ABANDONED
PICHER
OKLAHOMA

ABANDONED PICHER OKLAHOMA

THE MOST TOXIC TOWN IN AMERICA

REGINA DANIEL

AMERICA THROUGH TIME®
ADDING COLOR TO AMERICAN HISTORY

America Through Time is an imprint of Fonthill Media LLC
www.through-time.com
office@through-time.com

Published by Arcadia Publishing by arrangement with Fonthill Media LLC
For all general information, please contact Arcadia Publishing:
Telephone: 843-853-2070
Fax: 843-853-0044
E-mail: sales@arcadiapublishing.com
For customer service and orders:
Toll-Free 1-888-313-2665

www.arcadiapublishing.com

First published 2019

ISBN 978-1-63499-196-4

Typeset in Trade Gothic 10pt on 15pt
Printed and bound in England

INTRODUCTION

Picher Oklahoma will always have special place in my heart. It is where being an urban explorer started for me. It was 2014 and, to be honest, I had never even heard of Picher until watching a show about its history and today's current condition. This sparked my curiosity to visit this ghost town on more than one occasion. I went as a curious onlooker in 2014 but would return in 2019 as an experienced urban explorer. Over the span of my photos, I detail the decay of what the town had left to offer, as well as my growth as a photographer. In addition to learning another small chapter in American history, Picher also taught me, as a photographer, to photograph everything. Had I known then where being an urban explorer would take me, I would have documented so much more before it was gone for good. Another factor that adds to making this town so special to me is that Picher's story of abandonment differs from all the other places I have explored. When a school or business closes, life still maintains a level of normalcy except for going to a new job or school. However, with Picher, what was established to be a profitable mining town resulted in lives being uprooted and permanently effected by a long-term wake of environmental and physical devastation. The contamination is only the beginning of this disastrous and ongoing story.

Located in the most northeast corner of Oklahoma in Ottawa County, Picher has been labeled "the most toxic town in America"—and for good reason. After the discovery of crude ore in the early 1900s, Picher was established as part of the Tri-State Lead and Zinc District. Leasing the land for mining from the Quapaw Tribe of Oklahoma, the town started off as a modest mining camp for the workers. The start of World War I brought on the demand for lead and zinc for weapons and ammunition. With more than half of World War I's zinc and lead supply coming out of Picher, the population grew to nearly 10,000 residents just two years after the city's incorporation in 1918. Picher would reach its highest number of population

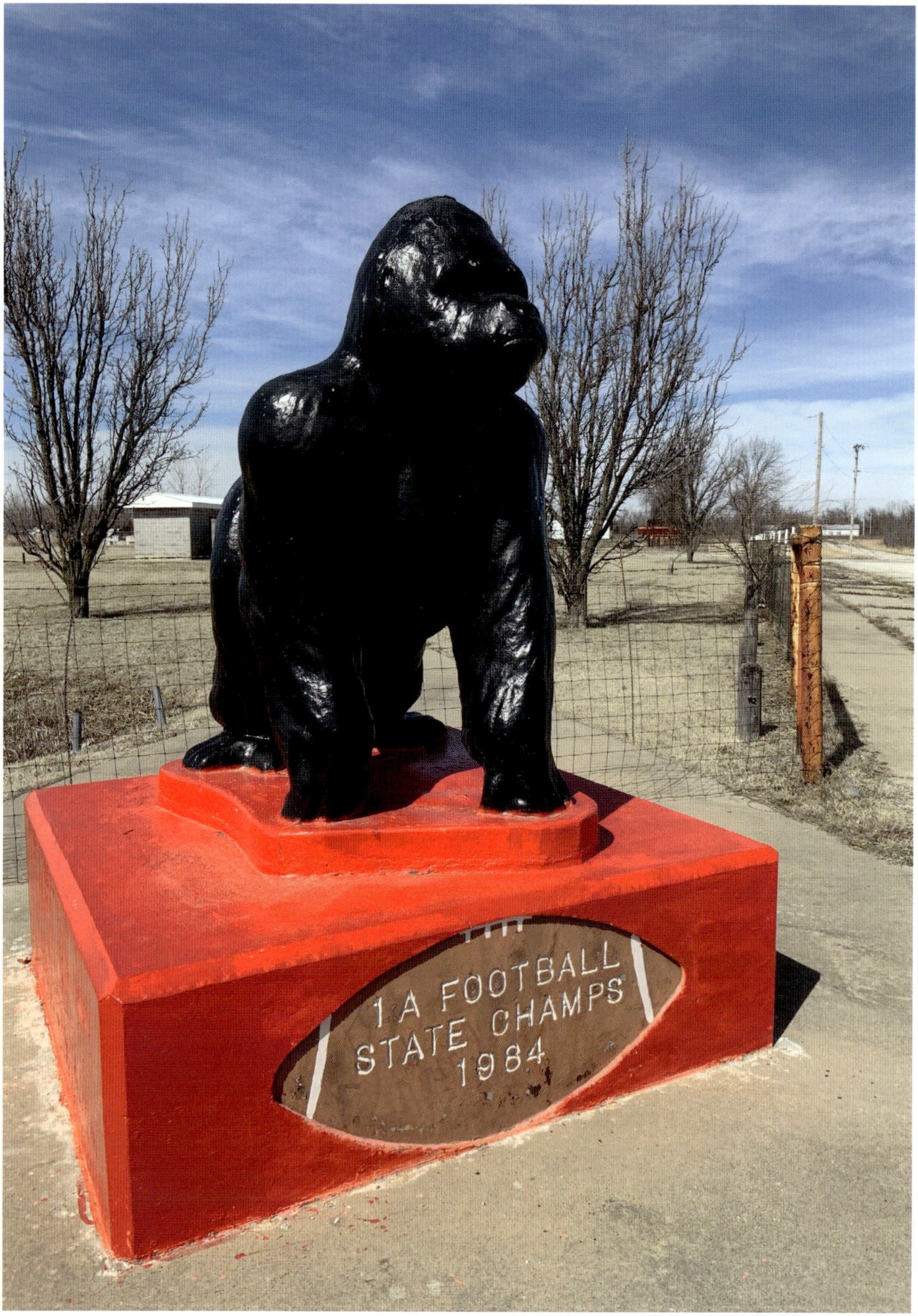

The Picher Gorilla, March 2019.

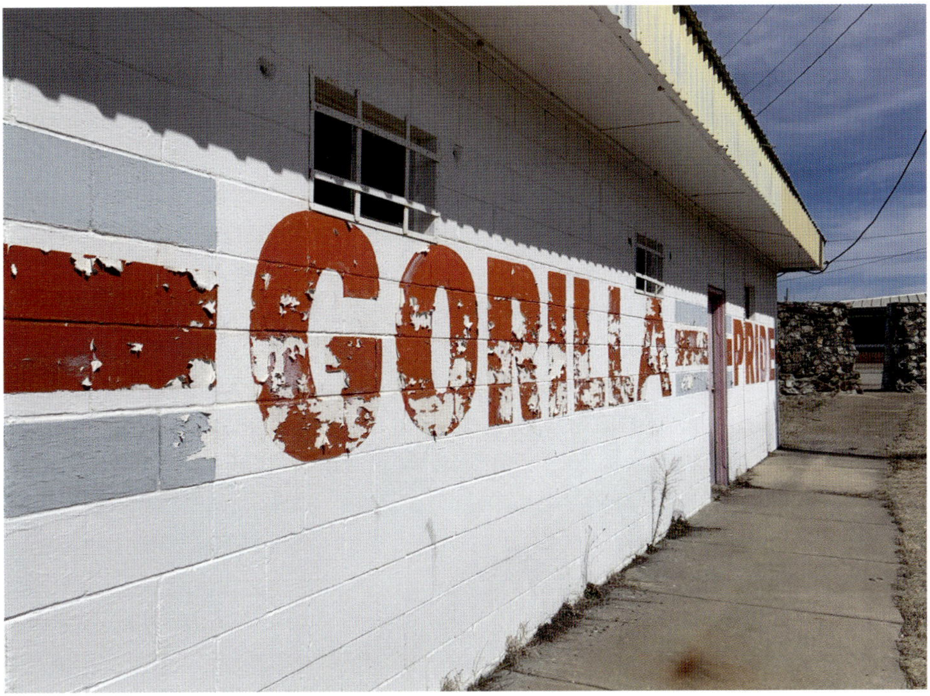

Peeling away Gorilla Pride, March 2019.

of slightly over 14,000 in 1926. Despite being the most profitable mine for Tri-State, Picher's population would decrease over the decades due to the ending of both World War I and World War II and the reduced demand for mining. After years of decline, in 1960, the town's population would drastically drop to 2,553, eventually leading to the closure of the mines in 1967. However, by this time, the damage had already been done. The myriad problems left behind resulted in a serious trickle-down effect on the land and its people, but that would not be known until several years later. The abandoned mines, now filled with lead-contaminated water, would eventually reach natural aquifers, spreading the lead poison into the town's water supply. The mountainous piles of Chat, a mining byproduct, still surround Picher, only adding to the pollution of the land and air, especially since the town wanted to be resourceful with all the chat by using it to pave roads, playgrounds, personal driveways, and parking lots. Part of this resourcefulness would lead to the contamination spreading to people's personal property as well as the mines and waterways. Another hazard that began to plague the town since the late 1960s was areas and homes above the abandoned mines have been swallowed up by sinkholes from the numerous collapsing abandoned mines. It was known in the late 1970s that the water in the mines had high levels of lead; however, it would not be tested and reported until 1980 that the town's natural aquifers were polluted and unsafe. Later that same year, the government started the Comprehensive Environmental Response Compensation and Liability Act (CERCLA), determining that Picher was a hazard and was placed on a National Priorities List, which determines governmental-funded cleanup and who gets it first. Finally, in September 1983, the mining area of Picher, known as Tar Creek, was deemed as a superfund project, in which multiple federal and local government agencies, including the Environmental Protection Agency (EPA), work together to begin the large scale clean-up efforts. Now the wheels were in motion to take care of the land and environment.

As for the individual effects, it was a 1996 study that put even more importance on having the area cleaned up. It was discovered that nearly 35 percent of the tested children did have an exceedingly high amount of lead in their systems—and that is just the children that were tested. Over a quarter of the town's children was at risk of a multitude of lifelong health problems. According to the Center of Disease Control (CDC):

> Lead poisoning can affect virtually every body system; it can damage a child's central nervous system, kidneys, and reproductive system. At high levels, lead can cause

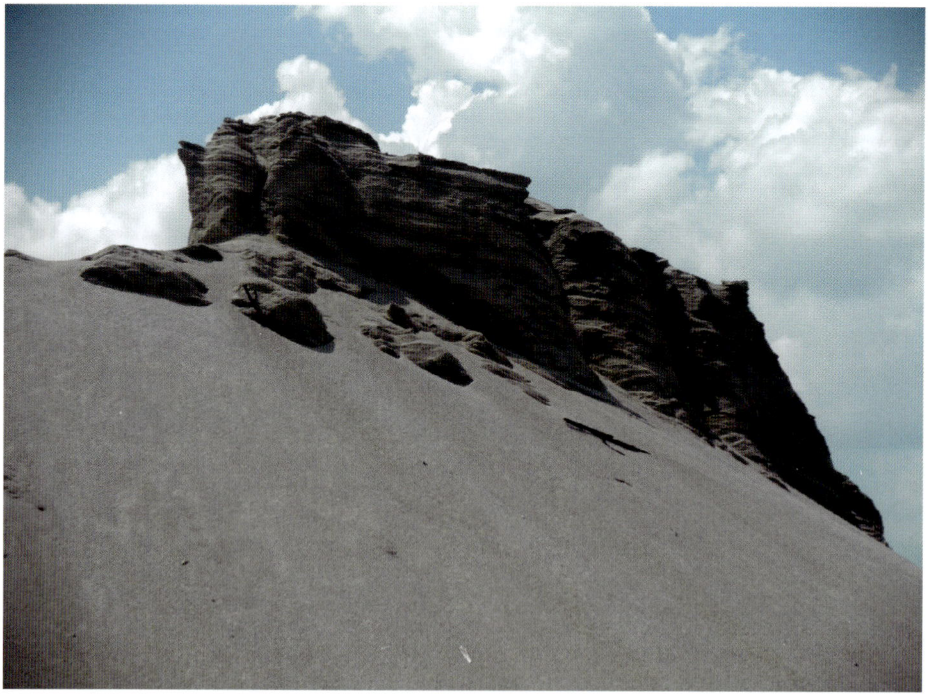

Close up of chat pile. Notice the striations from years of wind erosion, August 2014.

coma, convulsions, and death. Even low levels of lead in young children's blood can be harmful and can result in decreased intelligence, impaired neurobehavioral development, decreased stature and growth, and impaired hearing. Because childhood lead poisoning often has no distinctive clinical symptoms, it can go unrecognized.

I felt the need to use that direct quote instead of trying to put all or even some of those side effects into my own words because the CDC paints a difficult picture for just a child residing in that type of environment—think about the kids that played on the piles for hours every day and for how many years. There was no sugarcoating or paraphrasing those harsh realities. It was this study that put more importance on continuing to have the area cleaned up. The lead poisoning did not just effect the town's children, for the local expectant mothers, miscarriage rates increased more than double the national average. High lead levels in the blood is known to cause miscarriages, but should the baby be carried to term, those levels can and do cause physical damage to the baby *in utero*. Knowing what lead poisoning was doing to the woman and children of Picher, it would still take until 2006 for the government to start relocating the residents due to the increasing hazards to their physical well-being.

In addition to the many physical effects on the residents, the environmental aftermath is still currently going on. Today, there is at least 70 million tons of chat, blowing hazardous dust throughout the area. When tornados occur in the area, not only does debris get carried miles away, that lead and zinc fine powder also travels for miles all around. Those dustings may not cause the same level of damage, but it is still spreading contamination that can accumulate over time for wherever the dust lands. Animals are not immune to the pollutants that cover the town. Over 1,000 migratory birds have been found dead within the Picher area. It is speculated that all the bird deaths was caused by zinc poisoning. Being that zinc is in the chat and the birds were located in close proximity of the zinc in question, it my personal belief that this is all more than coincidence.

Although many of the residents moved away throughout 2006 and 2007, the horrible plight of this town does not stop there. For the remaining residents, May 2008 would add another unfortunate detail to Picher's bleak story. An EF4 tornado swept through Picher, leaving many of the residents injured, eight people died, and much more of the town in ruins. On top of all that, the government voted against sending any financial aid, due to the prior plans of relocating from the environmental hazards. Local government, however, did send aid and restored power for the local businesses and the nearly 1,600 people that still remained behind at that time, like

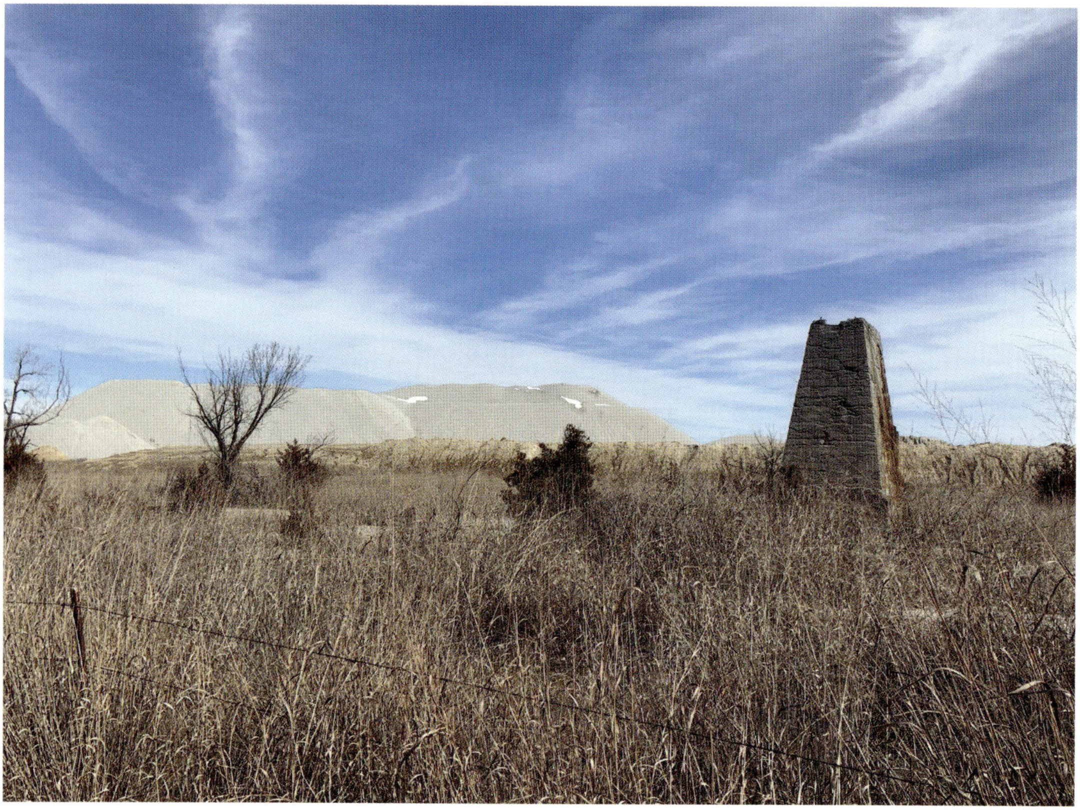

These chat piles have been sitting here since the 1960s, when the mining finally stopped in the Picher area, March 2019.

local man Gary Linderman, who owned and operated the only pharmacy in Picher. I mention Gary because he is subject of some debate and I think an important part of Picher's history. Some will say that he was the last resident of Picher; however, researched statistics and my own personal trips to Picher could argue otherwise. A resident, no doubt about that, but not the last.

Throughout 2009, locals would go on to see their post office and city hall close, another sinkhole take out another part of the town, and the last eleven seniors to graduate high school before transferring the remaining students to surrounding schools. Then, in 2011, demolition of a lot of the town started, tearing down empty and dilapidated businesses. All that was left was a small handful of buildings.

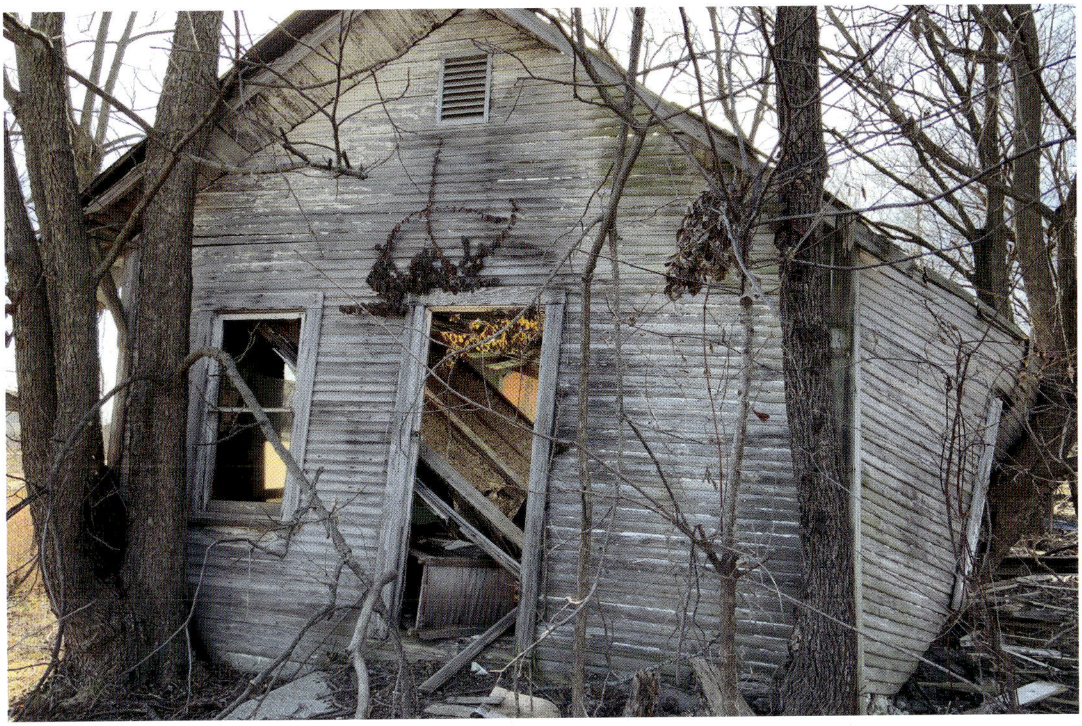

This house is so damaged, it is a surprise that the front is still standing, March 2019.

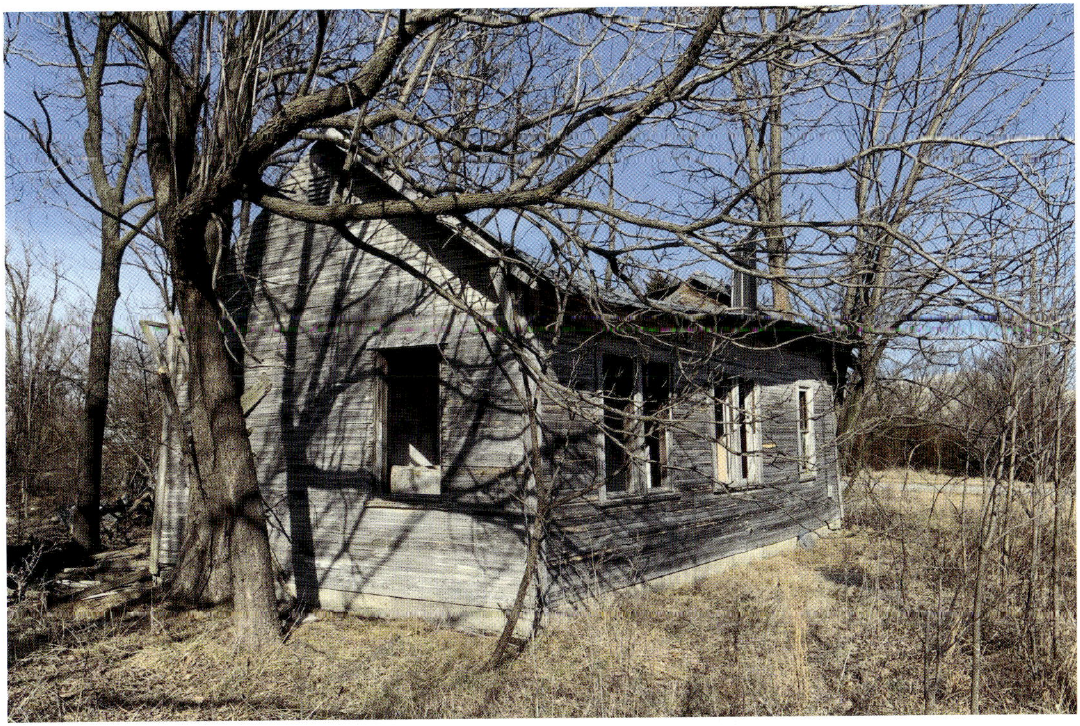

Like many of the remaining houses, the collapsed roof is just the start of the natural elements tearing down what was left abandoned, March 2019.

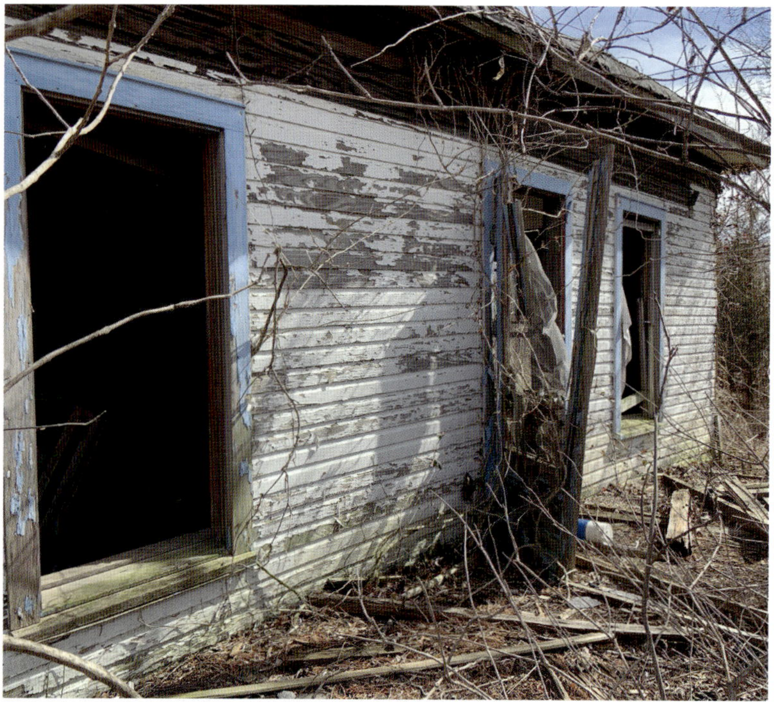

Despite missing windows and the front door, the screen door is surprisingly still hanging on, March 2019.

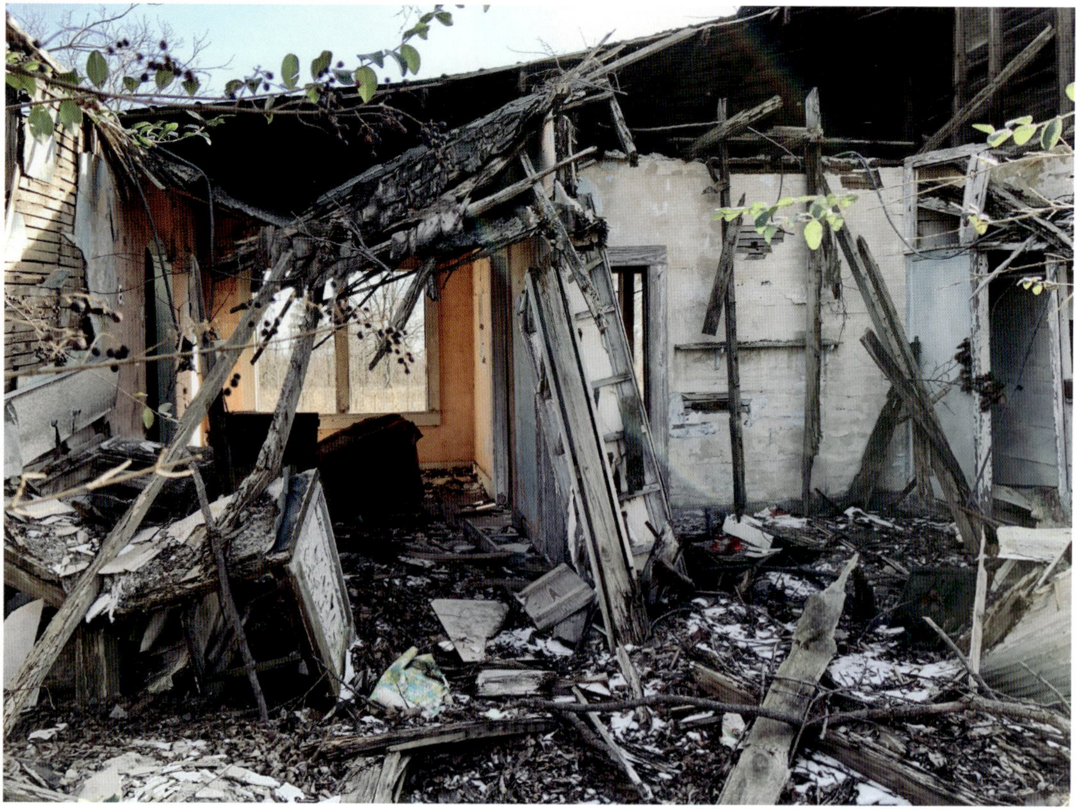

Side view of collapsed house, March 2019.

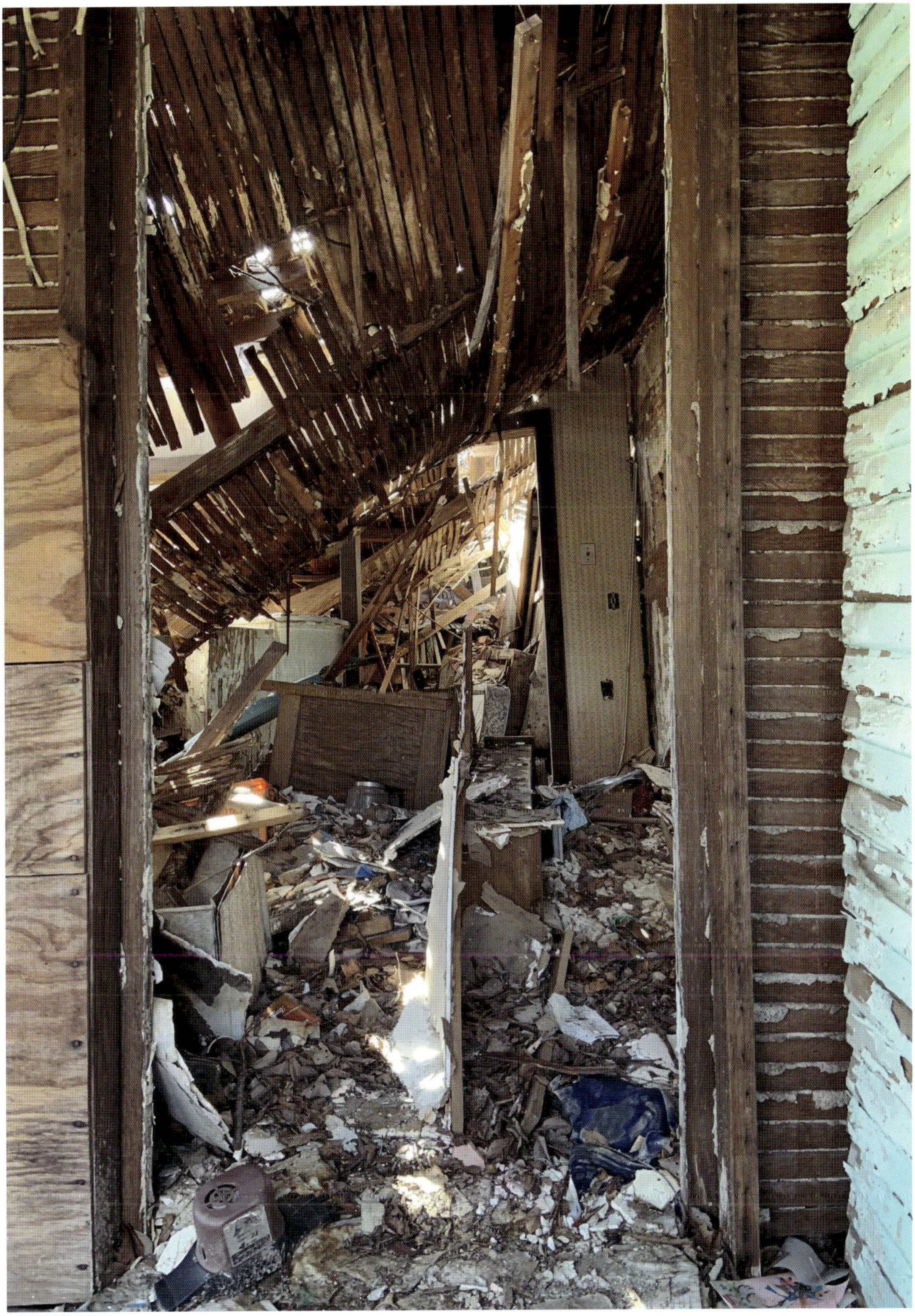

View inside a collapsing house, March 2019.

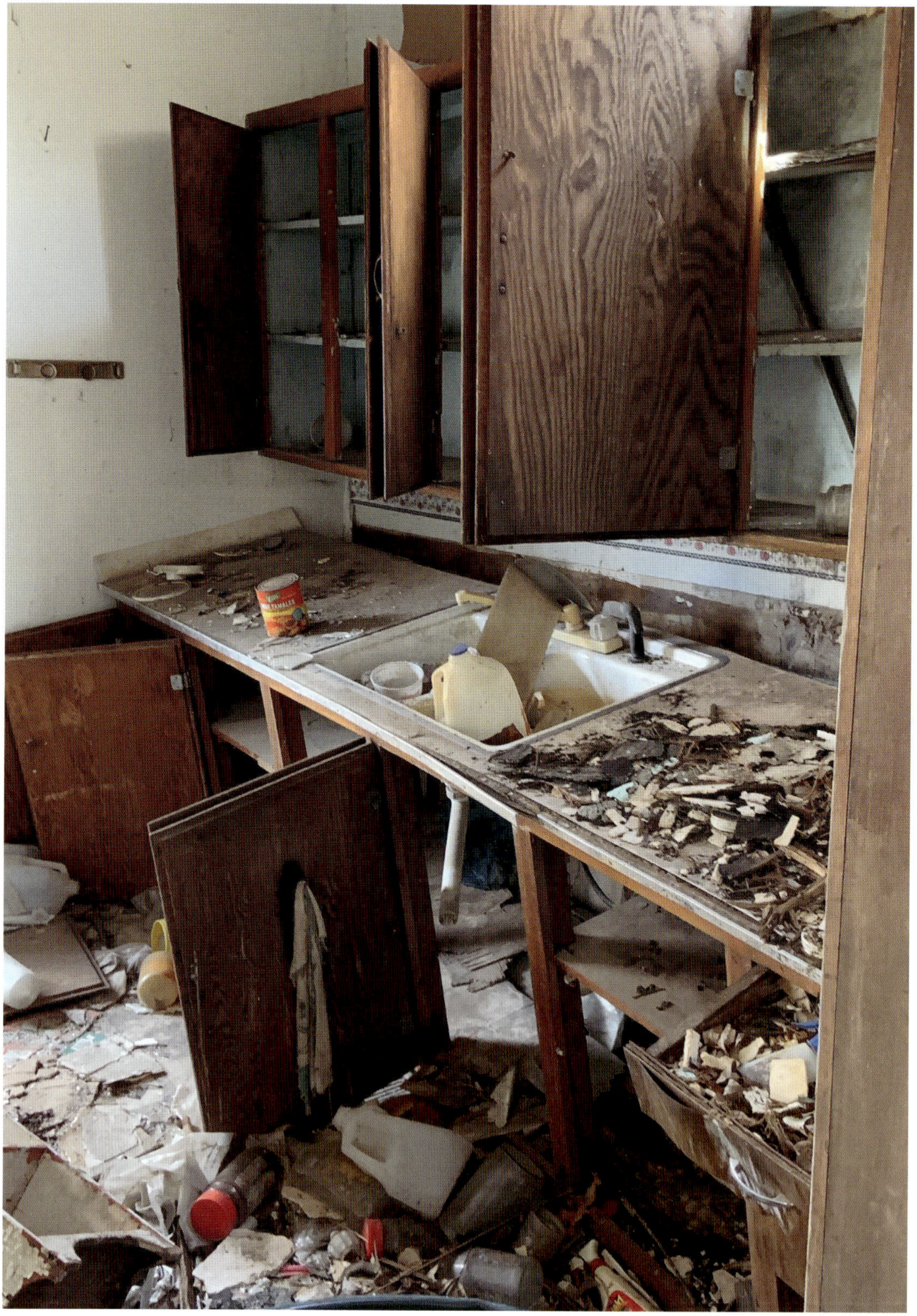

Kitchen left in shambles after house was abandoned, March 2019.

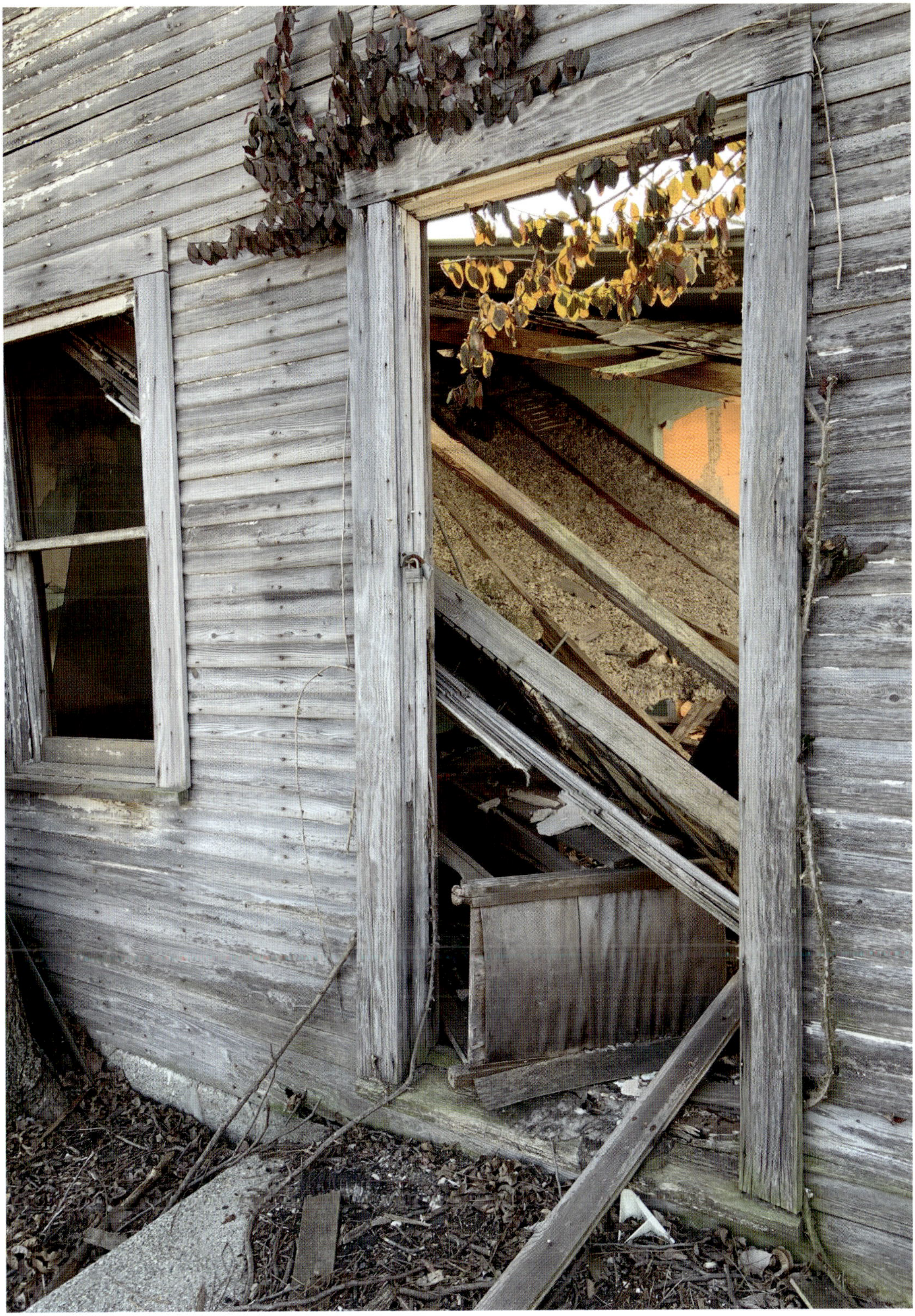

The damage is so much that you cannot even go through the front door, March 2019.

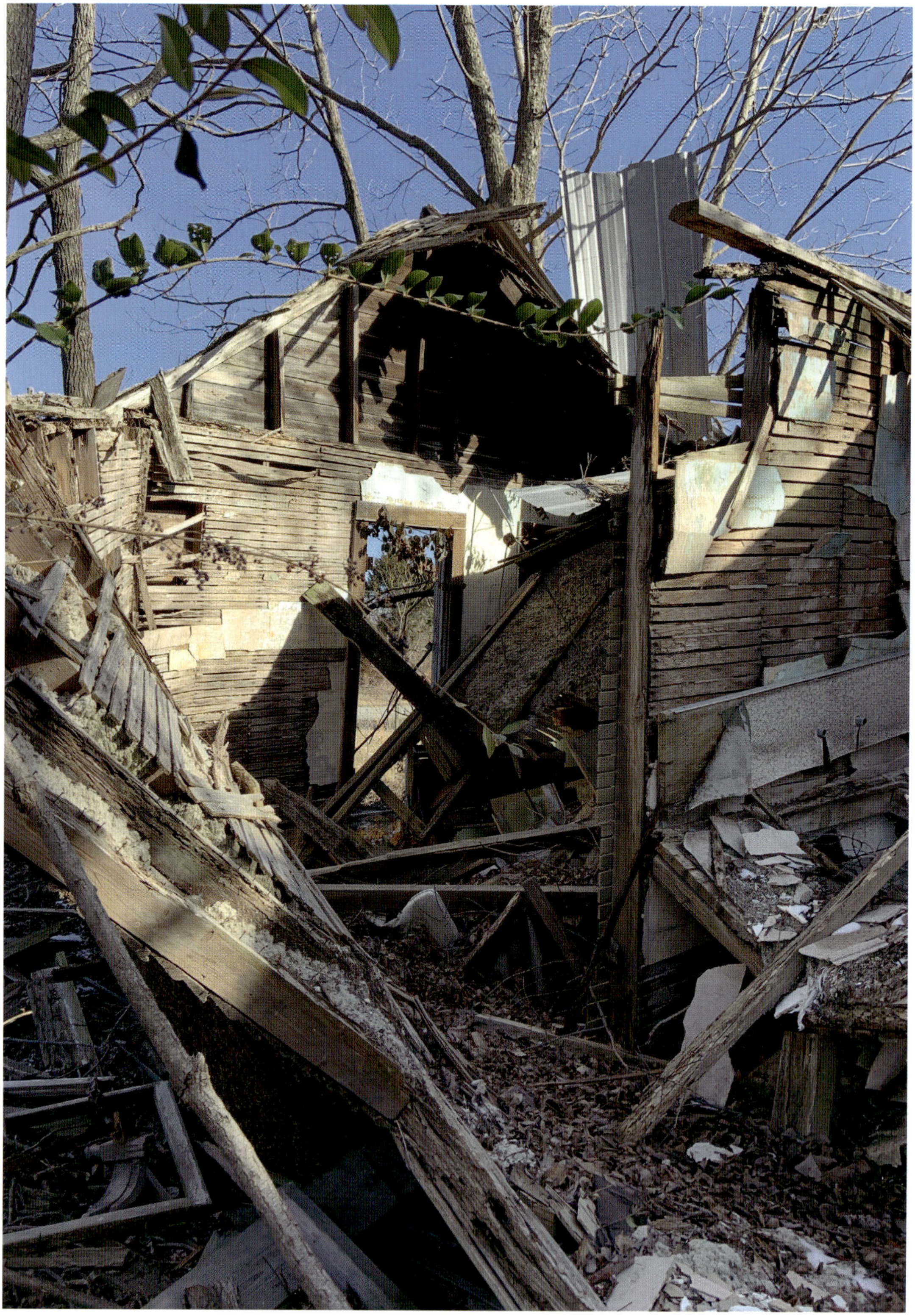

Full back view of collapsed house, March 2019.

ABANDONED PICHER, OKLAHOMA

The summer of 2014 is when I made my first trip down to Picher. As you enter town, the gargantuan chat piles are on both sides of Connell Avenue, the main road through town. The first building we encountered was the Picher Mining Museum. Although it was empty, the museum managed to stay completely intact. Walking through the multi-room building, there was no damage from vandals or looters, just big open empty rooms. The overgrowing plant life was just starting to grow on and up the walls inside the museum. The fireplace was in solid and good condition in the back room, and there was a small closet-sized walk-in fireproof safe in the back right corner of the museum. I am guessing that this was used for storing historical documents and smaller displays.

Just a couple more blocks down the road is where town begins. Greeting you is the Picher Gorillas water tower, standing tall in the parking lot between Linderman's pharmacy and a small slab home housing edition that consists of about twenty-five ranch-style duplexes. "KEEP OUT" was spray-painted all over the inside and outside walls of the duplexes, and all but one of those homes was completely gutted. All windows and doors had been removed. Standing there, you could hear the wind whistle through the shells of what used to be homes. The one unit that was not cleaned out was home to one of the few people that stayed behind and was still living there. I wanted to talk to him, however, him throwing knives into a spray-painted bullseye on the side of his house made me nervous about approaching him. I decided to let him be and continue on.

Moving on to the other side of the street remained a small strip of stores; a thrift shop that still had some clothes being displayed in the window, as well as a couple other closed up businesses. The last part of the strip was completely gutted down to the beams. In the back of that building, I found this old teddy bear, just sitting there. I only bring up the bear because it will go on to have another part in this story.

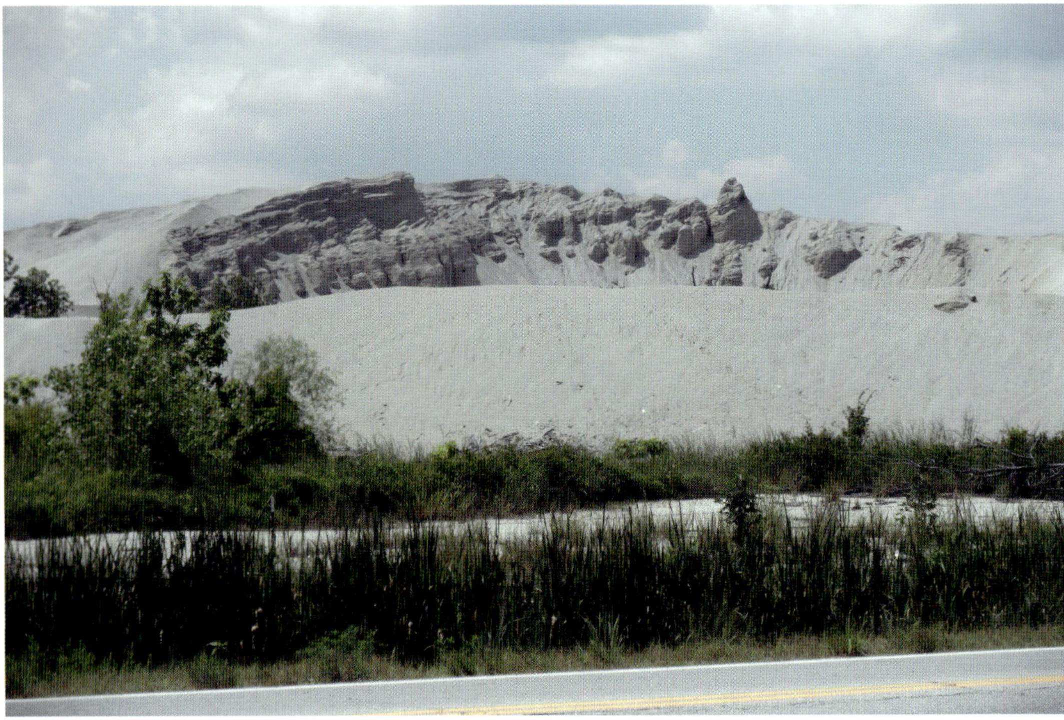

One of the many chat piles that surrounds the town of Picher, August 2014.

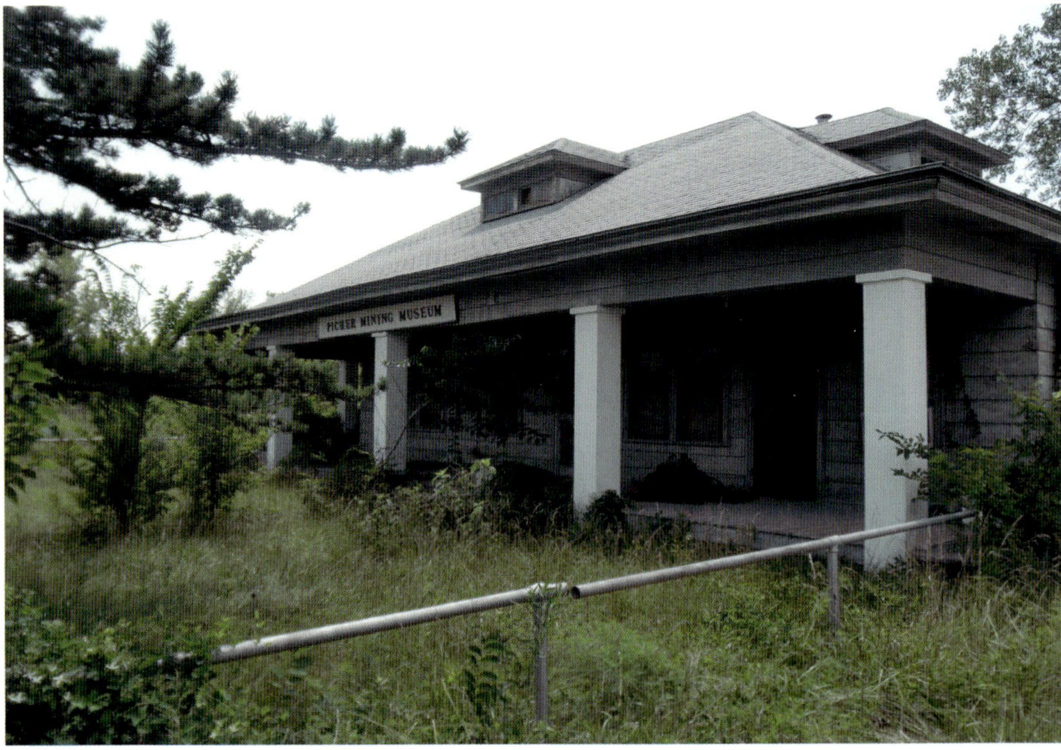

Picher Mining Museum in August 2014.

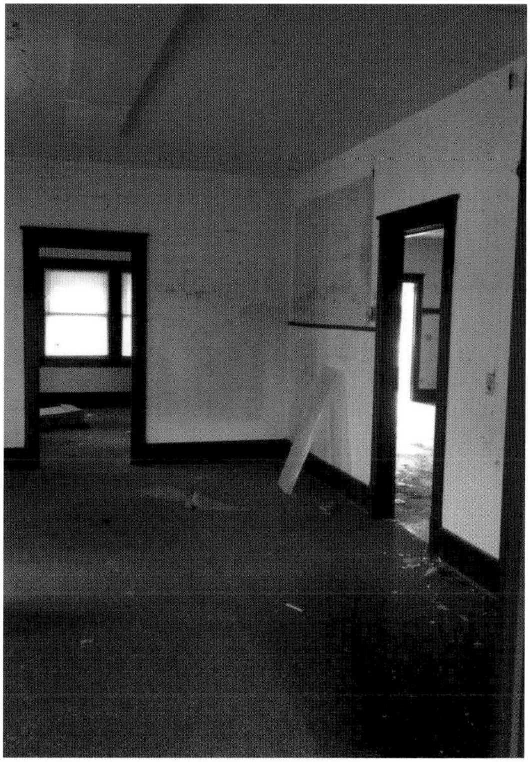

Rooms inside the Picher Mining Museum, August 2014.

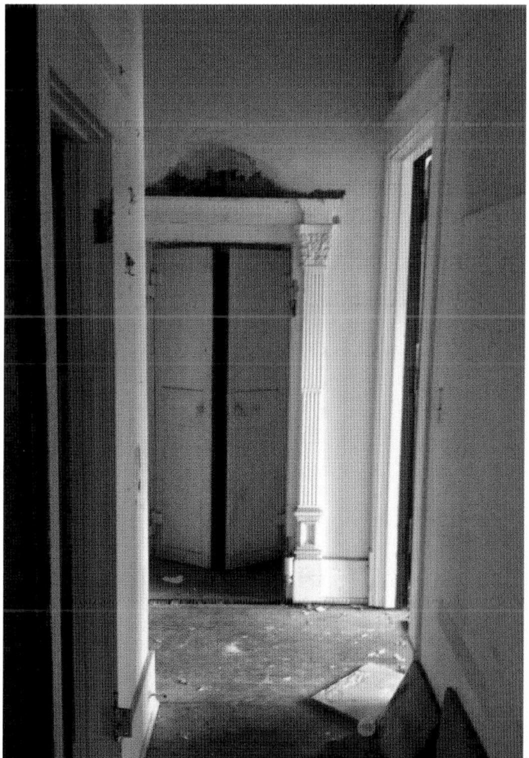

Hallway view to the walk-in fireproof safe inside the Picher Mining Museum, August 2014.

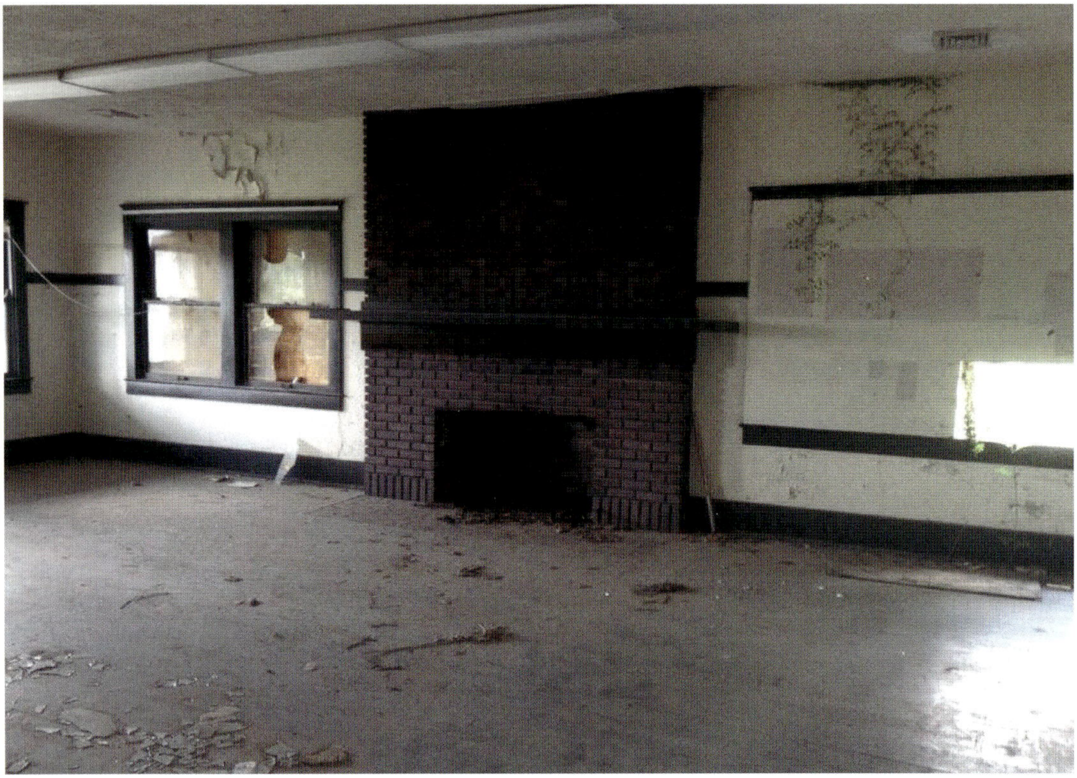

Fireplace in the back of the Picher Mining Museum, August 2014.

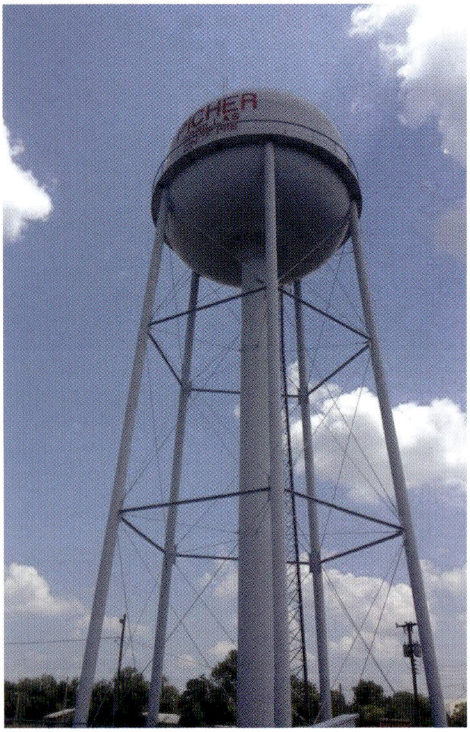

The Picher water tower in August 2014.

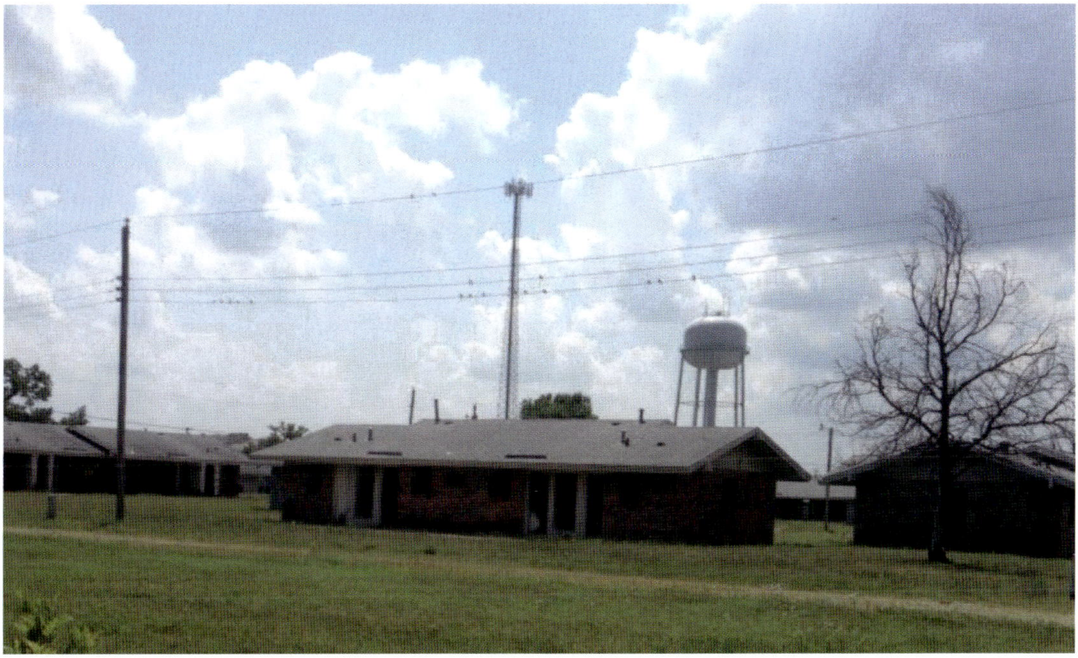

Ranch duplex complex and water tower in August 2014.

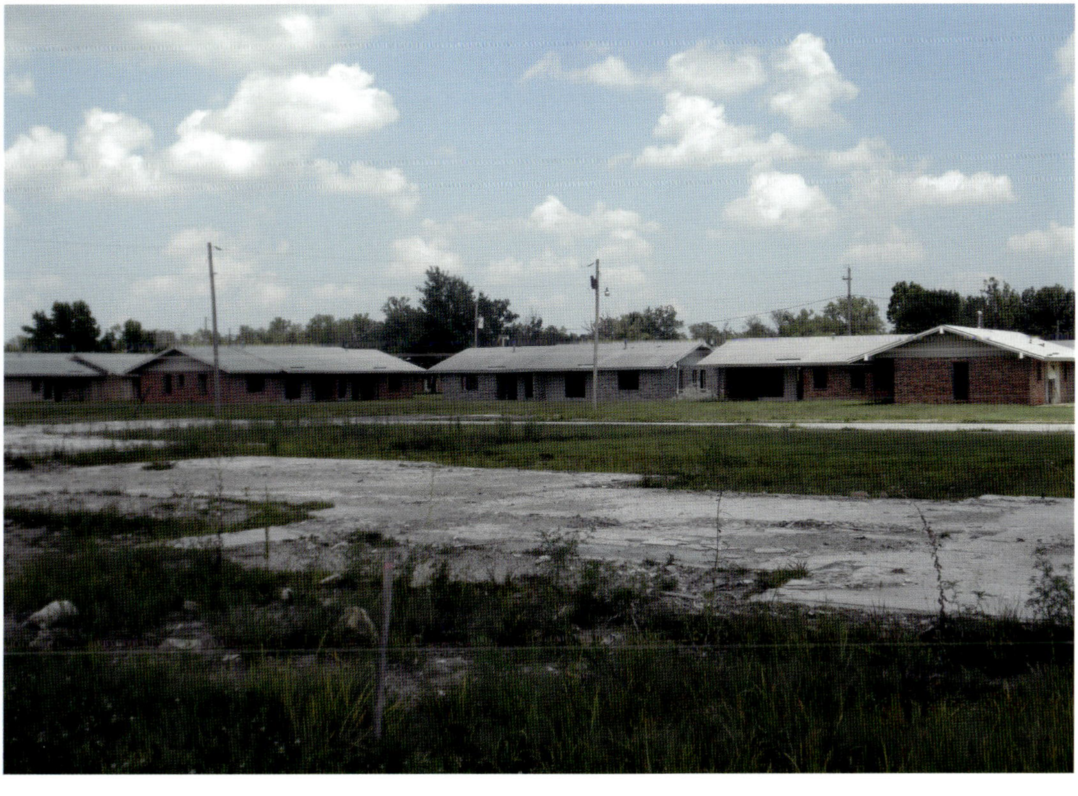

Duplex complex in August 2014.

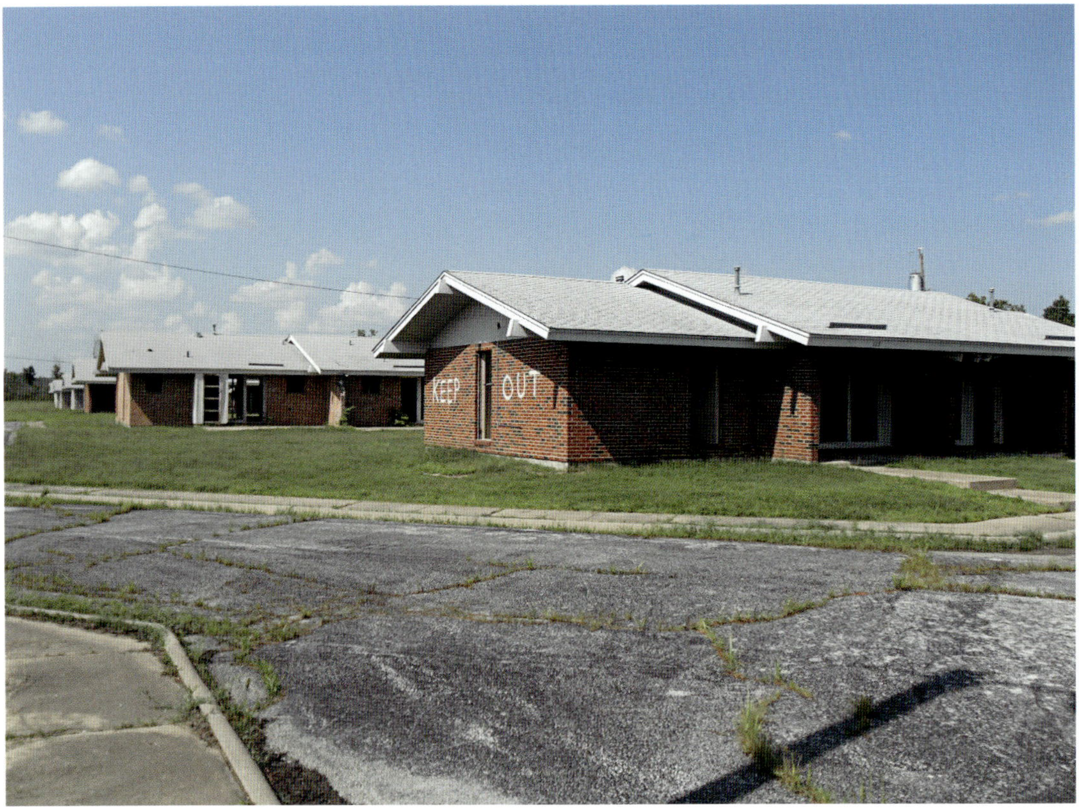

Duplexes with "KEEP OUT" spray painted on the sides, August 2014.

All those stores looked as if they had been closed up for a long time—spider webs in the windows and thick dust settled on the window ledges. What was once someone's bread and butter was now closed up and left as it was the day it closed—however many years ago.

Directly behind the small storefronts was a small grouping of houses. Like much of the town, these houses were also just left open for anyone to walk through freely. Personal belongings scattered the floors, furniture still sat in the living room, and there was even a couple of canned goods still sitting in the cupboards.

One of those in the grouping was a mobile home with some furniture and belongings inside. It was easy to see all that, including the bright green kitchen, because the walls that cover the frame were all gone, just leaving it stripped down to the beams. Looking at it, you would think it was one heavy gust of wind from falling apart, but the craftsmanship of this trailer would outlast a good portion of the town.

On the opposite side of Connell Avenue, by the city park, is the Picher Gorilla mascot statue. He was a bit dusty and faded, but the 1984 State Football Champs moniker could still clearly be read. Interesting side note to the gorilla statue: when the school was closed in 2009, the town held a public auction for the reusable school property, in which the statue was up for sale. Dave Marlin beat out three other bidders to purchase the gorilla for $2,500. It was delivered to its new home 130 miles away in Conway, Missouri. It was not stated when or why the statue was then brought back to where it sits today. Maybe Dave felt it needed to be back home where it belongs. The park behind the statue was overgrown at the time and was blocked off from anyone going in there.

Besides the big rusty engine and public restroom sitting in the middle of the park, there was not any remaining playground equipment. Driving around some more, I found the elementary school building along with the track and stadium. At this time, there was an active sheriff's station next door to the school, so getting into the school was not an option this time. The stadium seating had all been removed and someone was maintaining the track area. The Coke scoreboard was still standing at the end of the track and the concession stand building still had the Picher-Cardin All State Honor Roll names and red gorillas painted all around the building.

Going down "A" Street from the school was the big white Christian church. Still standing, it did take some damage from weathering and the 2008 tornado. The porch canopy had fallen off, partially blocking the front door. The interior was not nearly as damaged as the outside, but then again, there was not much in there to get damaged. I regretfully did not get any photos of the inside of the church.

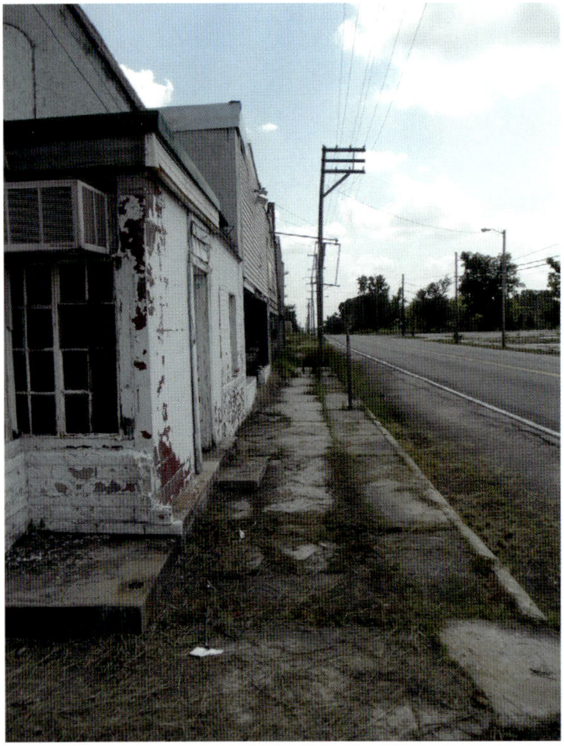

Left: Small strip of storefronts on Connell Avenue, August 2014.

Below: Second store from the corner. Painted flowers can still be seen, but the business name is now covered with a board, August 2014.

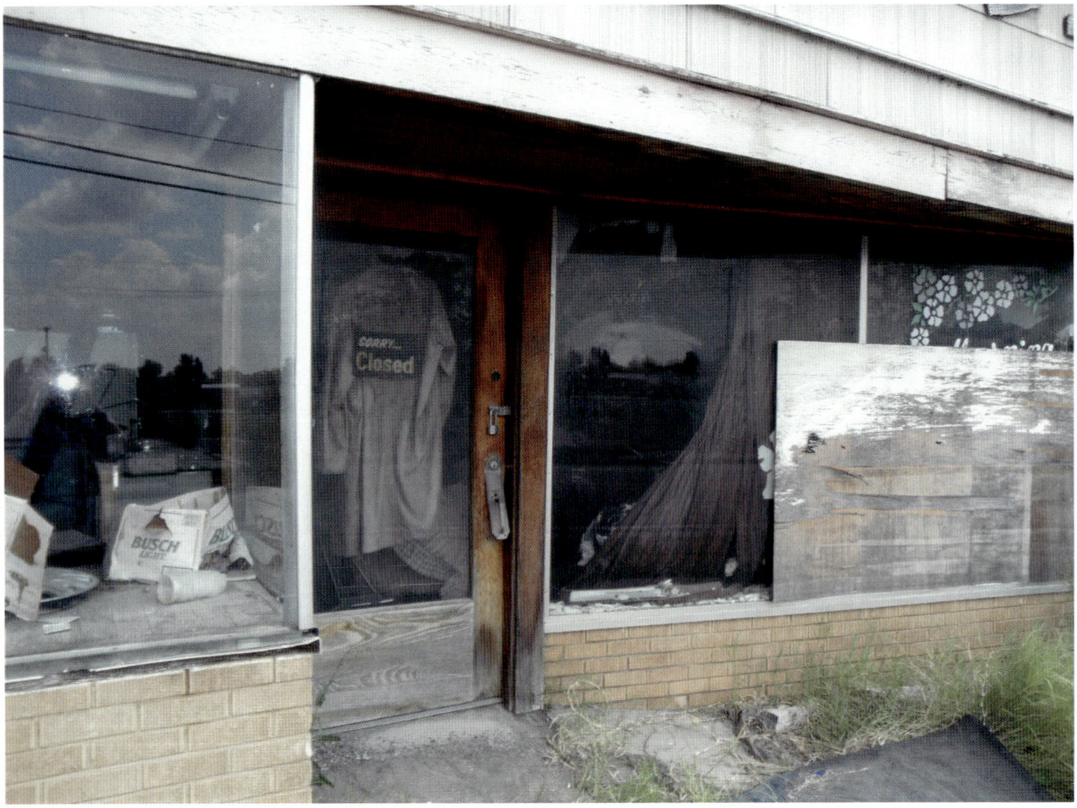

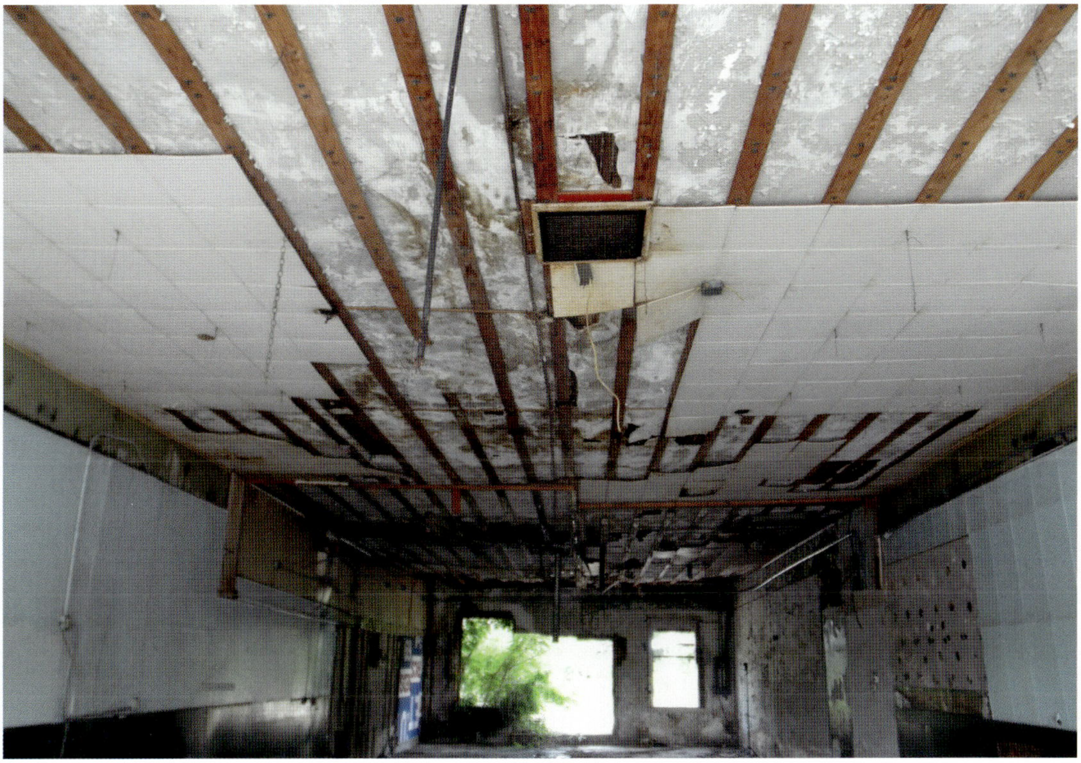

Last store in the strip of stores. This unrecognizable business has been stripped down to just beams and bare walls, August 2014.

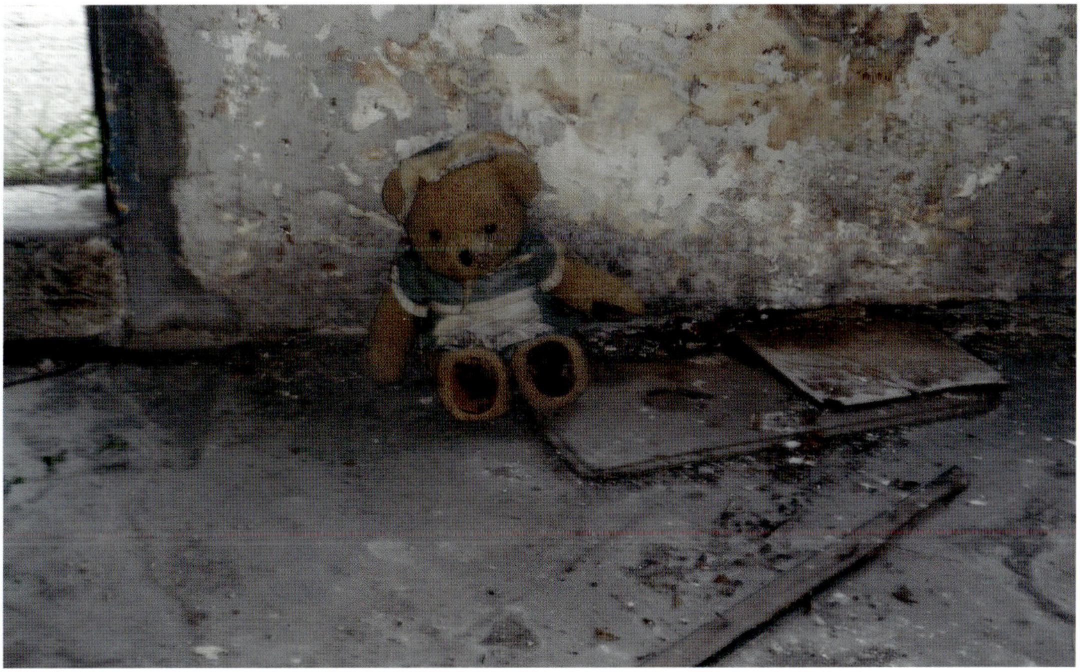

Teddy bear sitting at the back of the last store in the strip of stores, August 2014.

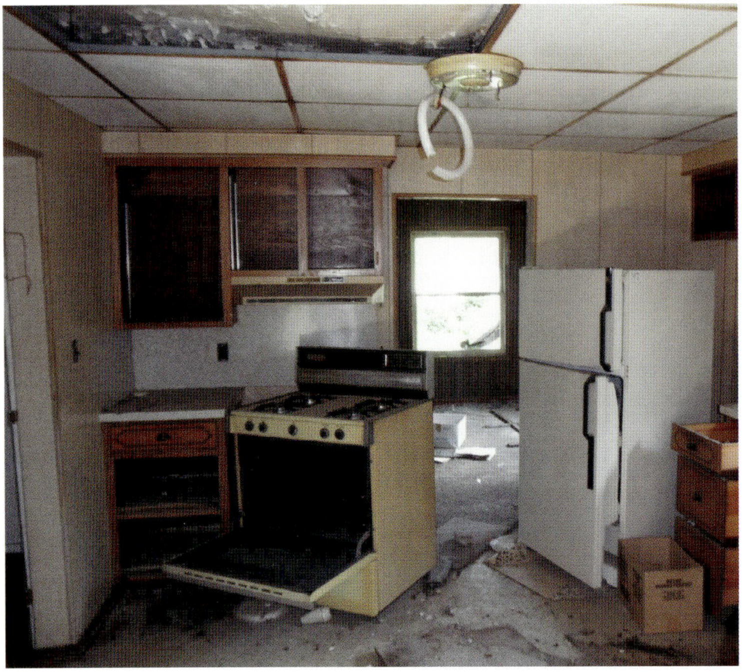

Kitchen in one of the houses located behind the strip of stores, August 2014.

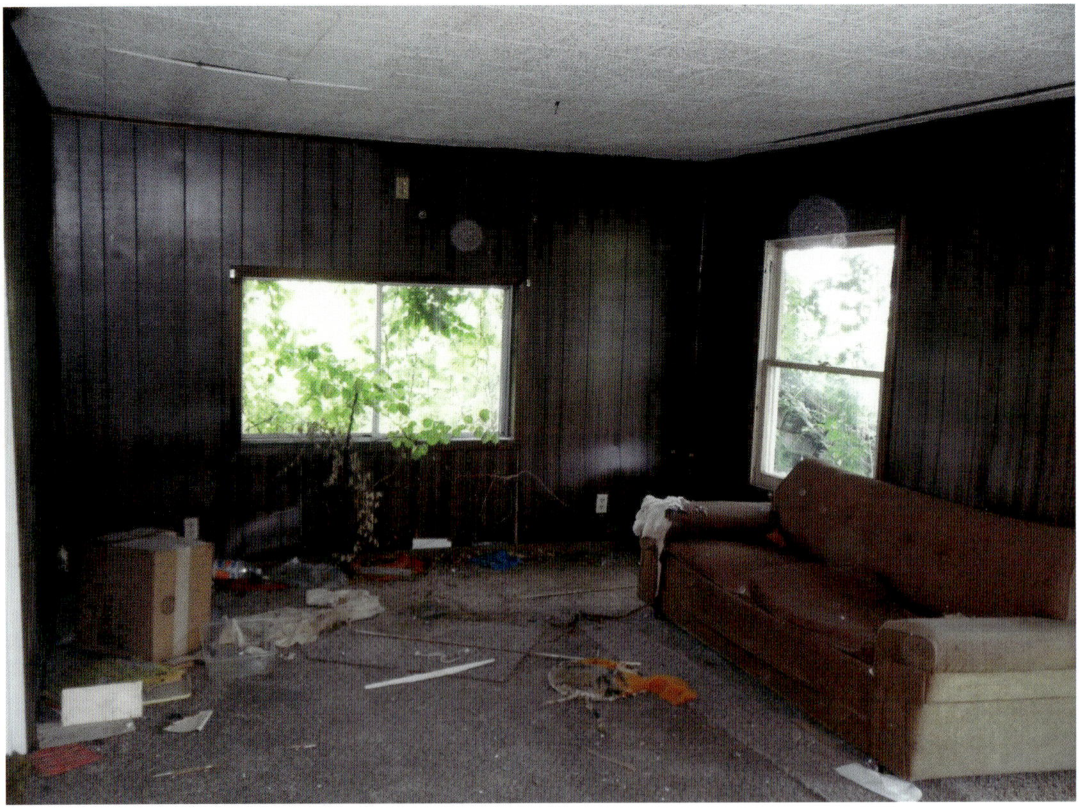

Next room over from the kitchen, the couch still sits in the living room of a house behind the strip of stores, August 2014.

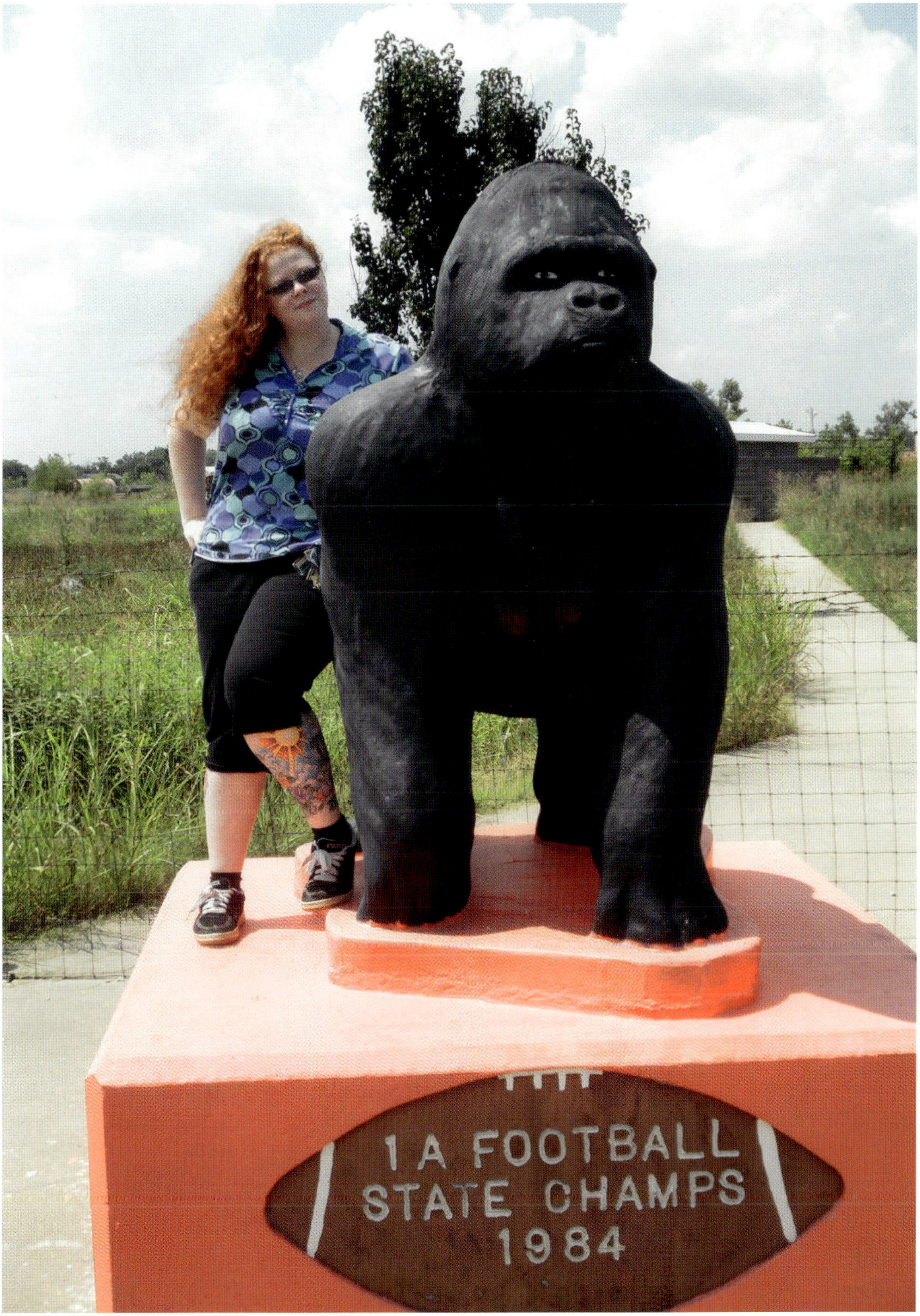

Regina and the Picher Gorilla statue in August 2014. (*Photo credit: Christopher Daniel*)

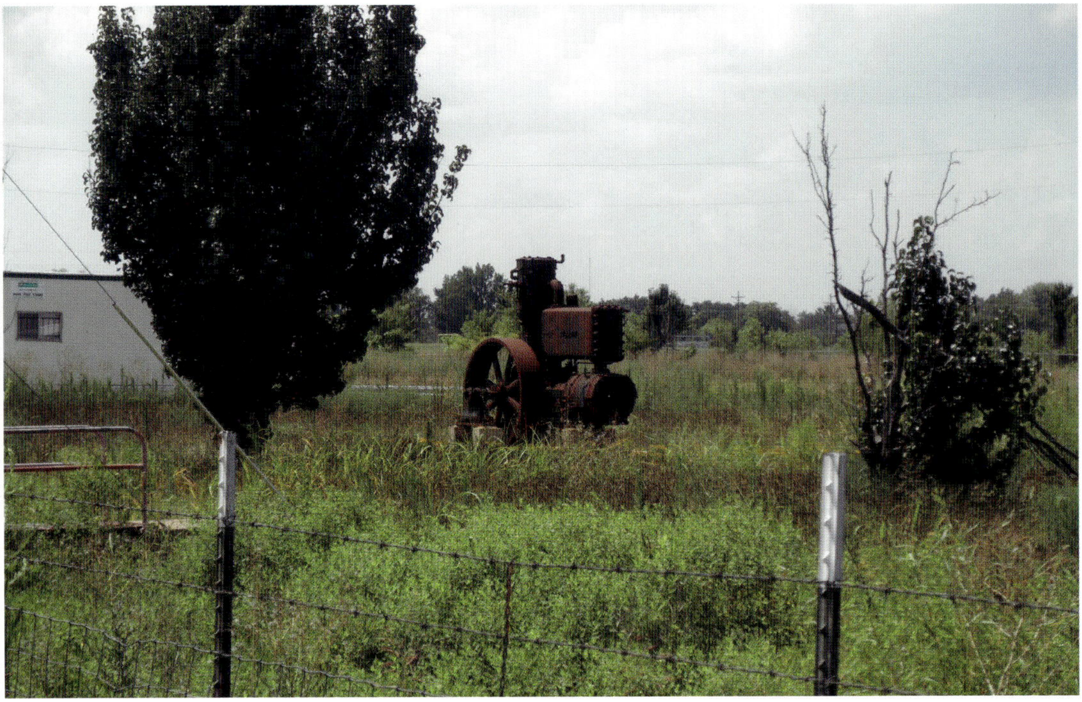

Big rusty engine sitting behind the gorilla statue in the city park, August 2014.

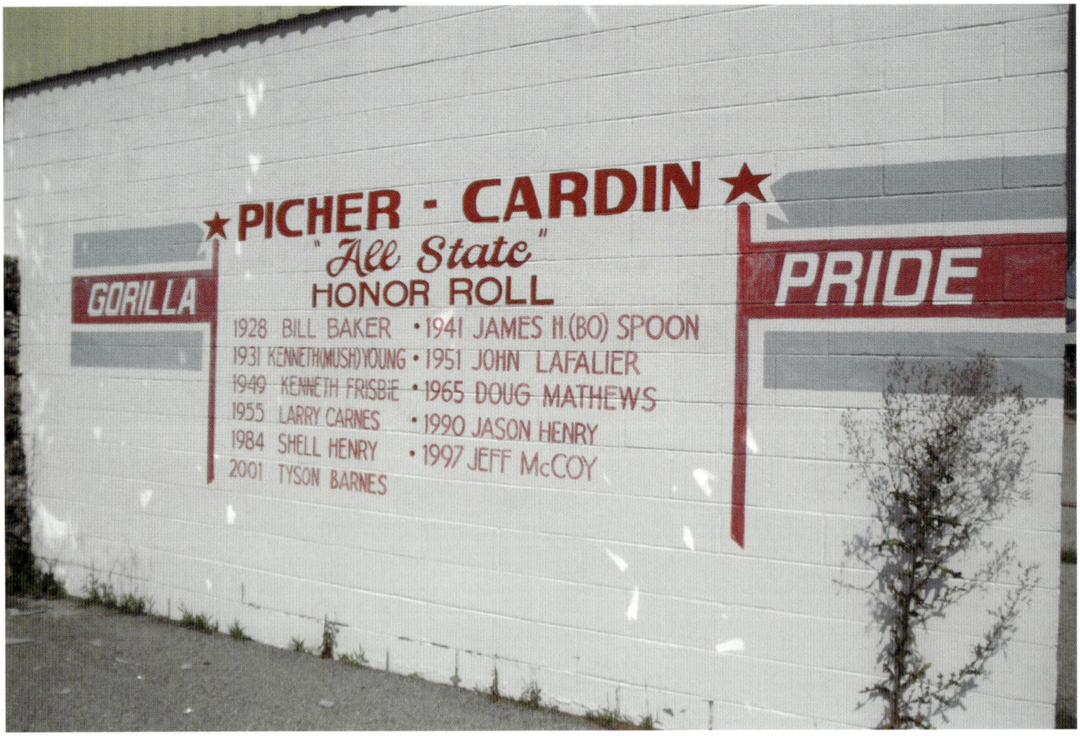
PICHER - CARDIN
"All State"
HONOR ROLL
GORILLA
PRIDE
1928 BILL BAKER
1931 KENNETH(MUSH)YOUNG
1949 KENNETH FRISBIE
1955 LARRY CARNES
1984 SHELL HENRY
2001 TYSON BARNES
•1941 JAMES H.(BO) SPOON
•1951 JOHN LAFALIER
•1965 DOUG MATHEWS
•1990 JASON HENRY
•1997 JEFF McCOY

The Picher-Cardin All State Honor Roll painted on the side of the school's fieldhouse/concession stand building, August 2014.

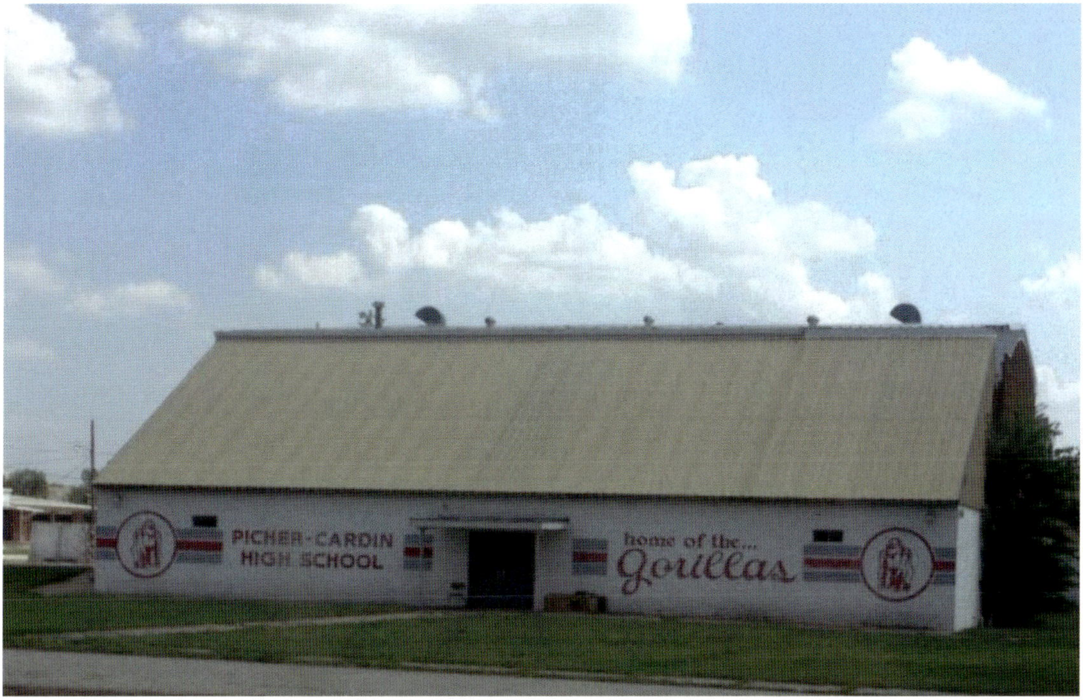

Front view of the school's fieldhouse/concession stand building, August 2014.

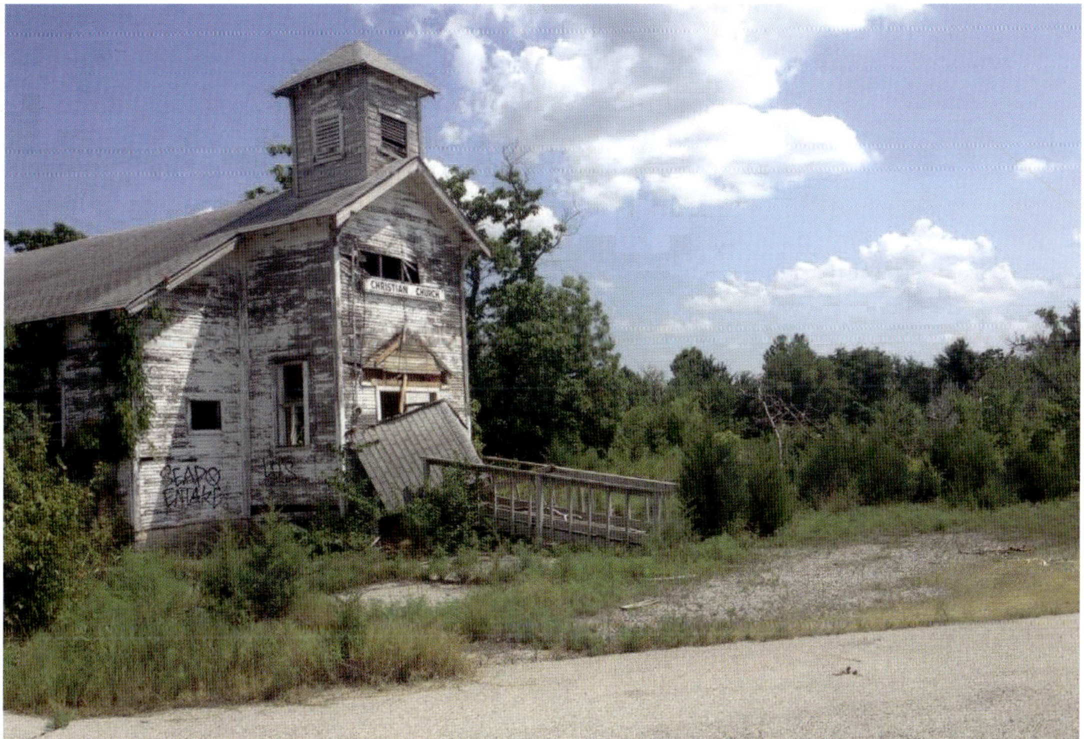

The Christian Church of Picher in August 2014. Unfortunately, it was burned down in 2017.

Moving along through town, there are many areas that are overgrown plots of land where house foundations lay in rows. Some of those foundations still had tiles glued to the concrete, peeling and faded from years of weathering. I imagine that back in the day, these areas were nice residential neighborhoods. Modest-sized homes with little yards, all aligned to make what was hoped to be a growing neighborhood. Now these concrete slabs serve as headstones for the memory of what used to be a home. At this point in 2014, it was estimated that Picher still had approximately ten residents remaining and driving around, you could see signs of life from those remaining residents. Cars in driveways, maintained lawns and landscaping, and one house even had an above-ground pool. Despite seeing all these signs of life, the town was eerily quiet and a general feeling of uneasiness, as if I was being watched. I went into this trip knowing some history and status quo, but I never expected the post-apocalyptic vibe that Picher put off. Records from 2015 indicate that the population had dropped to zero; however, when I returned in 2019, it appeared as if it had gone from the previous population in 2014 of ten to a few more. The exact number could not be located, but based off the number of lived-in-looking houses and people seen, I would say that number is now fifteen to twenty.

Unfortunately, on my first trip to Picher, I was merely a curious onlooker wanting to see the aftermath of when mining goes bad, so I did not take the number of photos that I would when I went back for the second visit. I did manage to photograph a couple of places that would not be there the next time—although, that would not happen for another five years.

On the return trip in early 2019, there was still many trucks and eighteen wheelers going through Picher, but that would not be enough to save the gas station diner that sat right at the Kansas and Oklahoma state line. It was completely gutted out, but the vintage metal V-shaped carport was still over where the gas pumps used to be.

It is not even a block before the old familiar chat piles start coming into view. They looked the same as they had before, but I cannot say the same for the mining museum. A year after my first visit, someone had set fire to the museum. Not knowing it had been set on fire, I nearly drove by what was left of the museum. The whole building was burned down, minus the front porch pillars, the back room brick fireplace, and fireproof walk-in safe. It was never disclosed as to if the arsonist was ever caught.

Other places in town, however, had not changed. The steadfast water tower still stands tall, displaying the Picher name. The ranch duplex complex looked as it did five years ago, except for the sheriff's station, which was previously next to the school and track, was now located in a couple of the renovated duplexes.

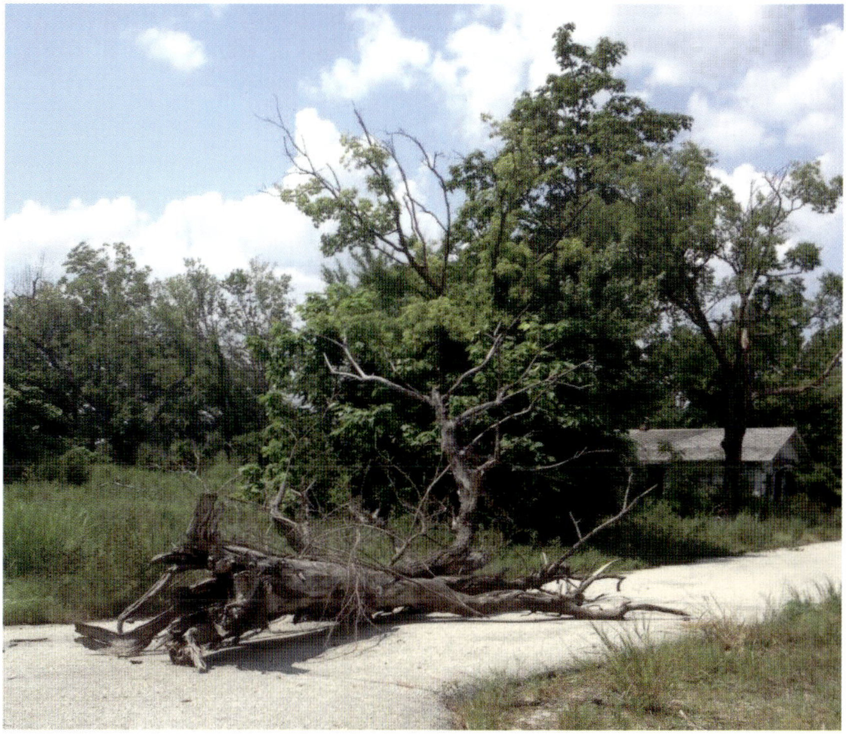

Fallen tree blocking the road in a residential area, August 2014.

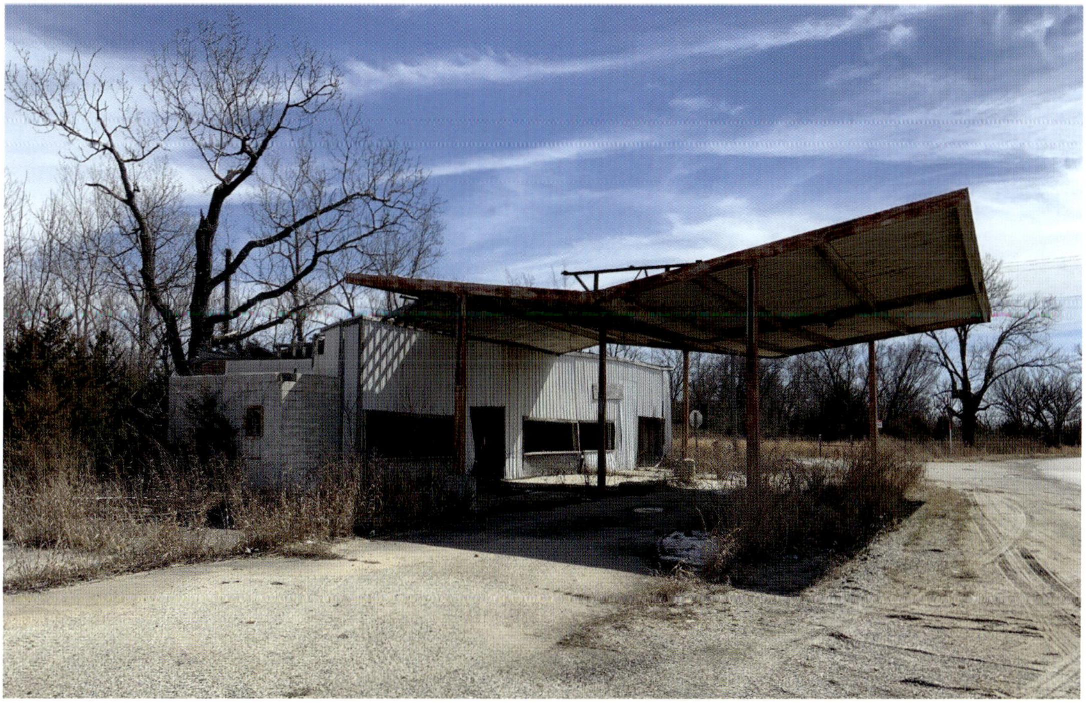

The twenty-four-hour gas station diner that sits right on the Kansas and Oklahoma state line, just a couple blocks outside of Picher. View from the Kansas side looking into Oklahoma, March 2019.

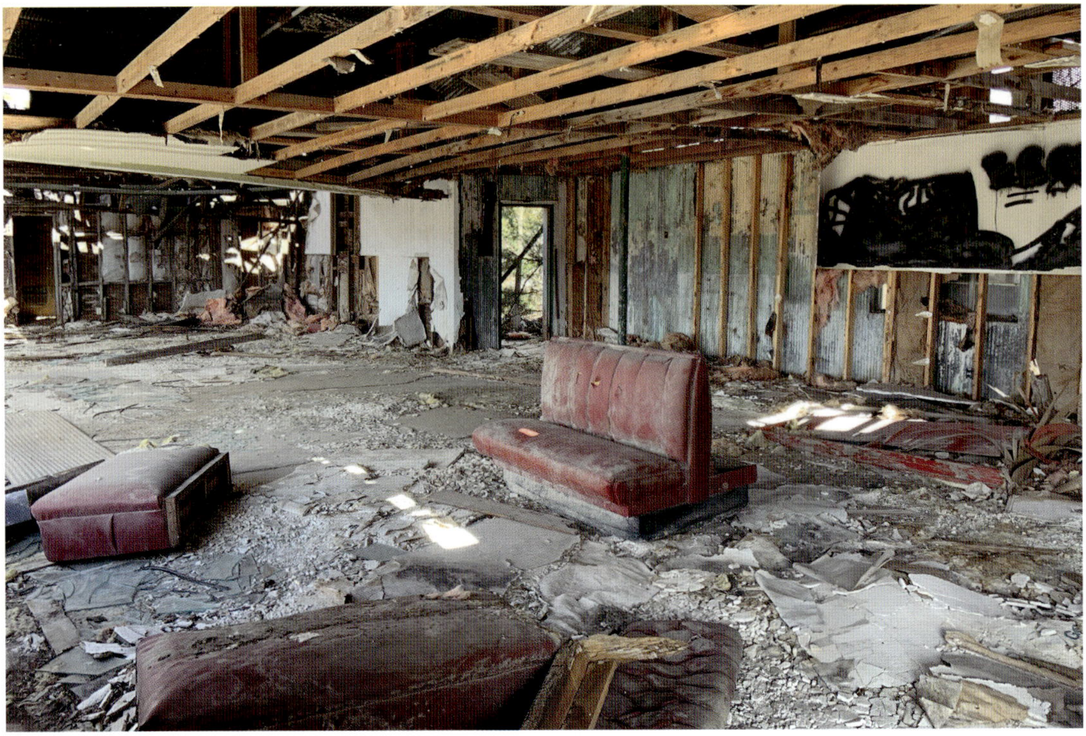

Inside the twenty-four-hour gas station diner, March 2019.

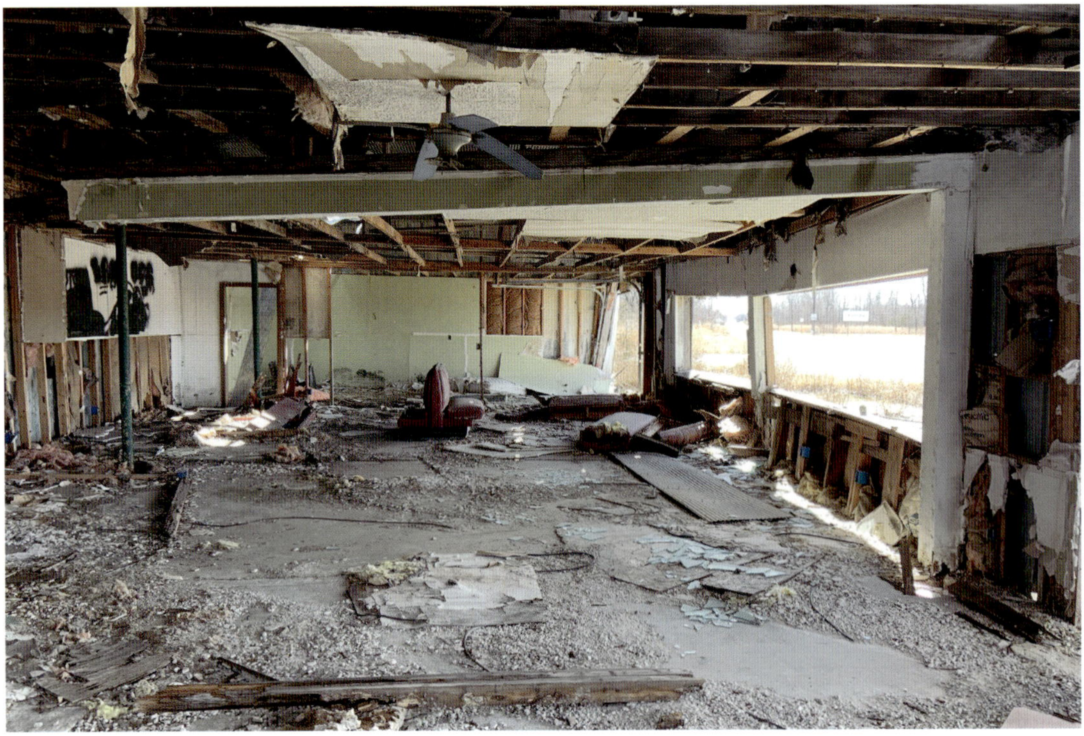

Inside the twenty-four-hour gas station diner, March 2019.

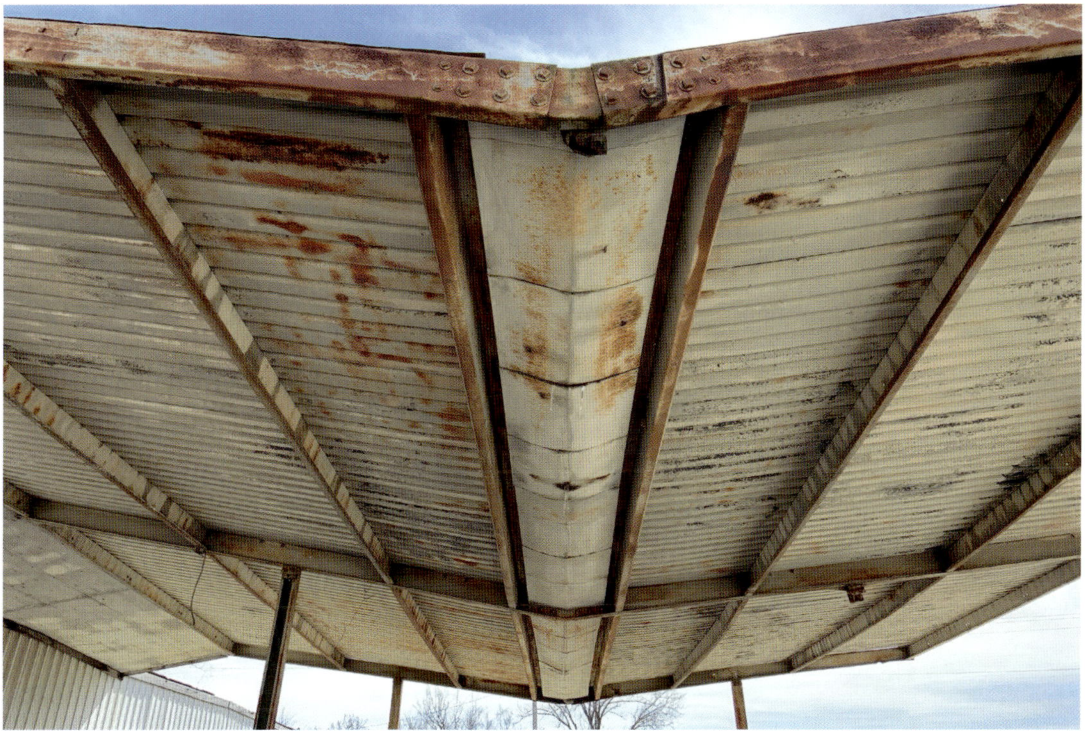

The V-shaped carport over the gas pumps at the twenty-four-hour gas station diner, March 2019.

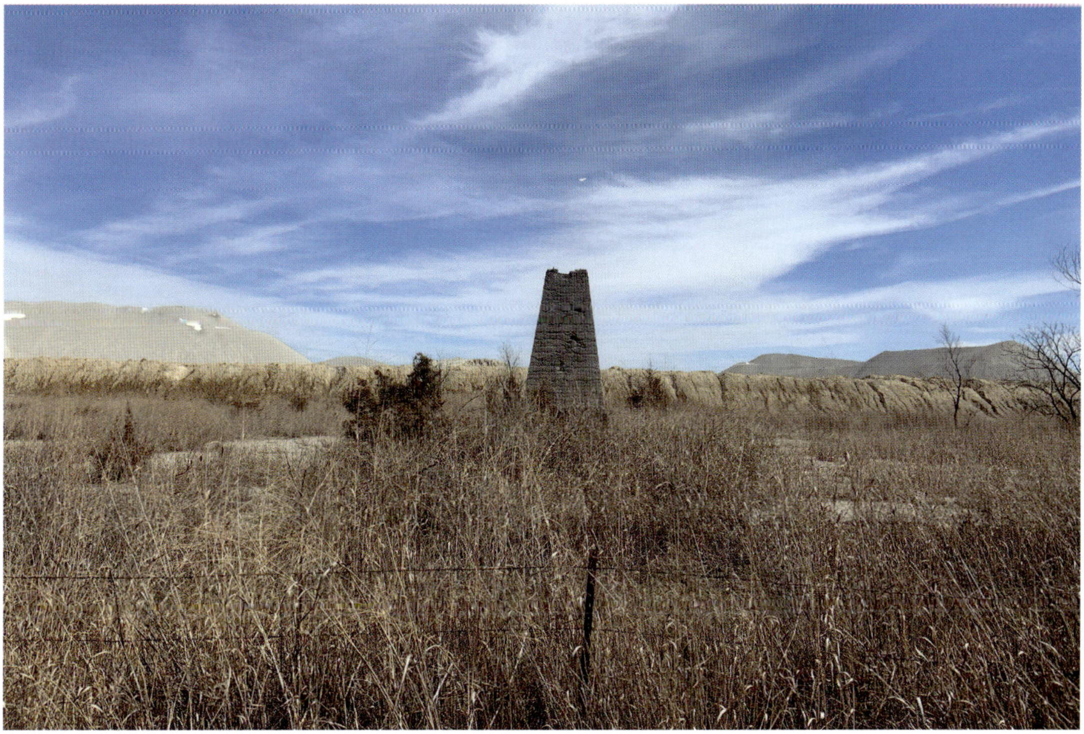

Some of the chat piles as you drive into Picher, March 2019.

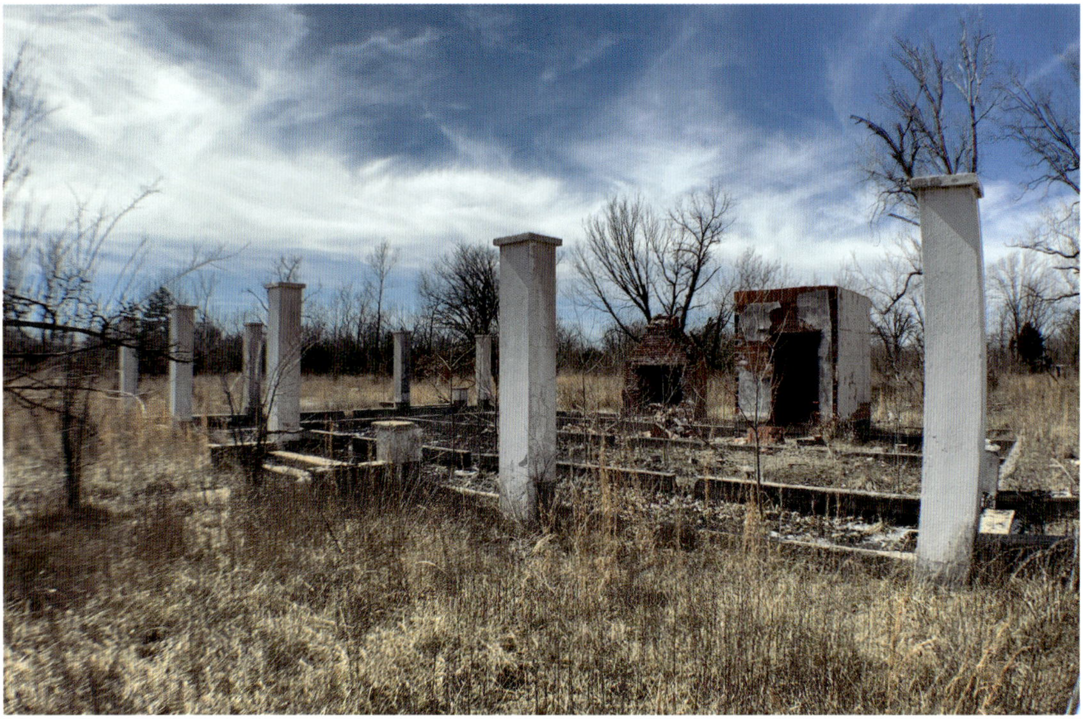

After being set on fire in 2015, this is all that remains of the Picher Mining Museum, March 2019.

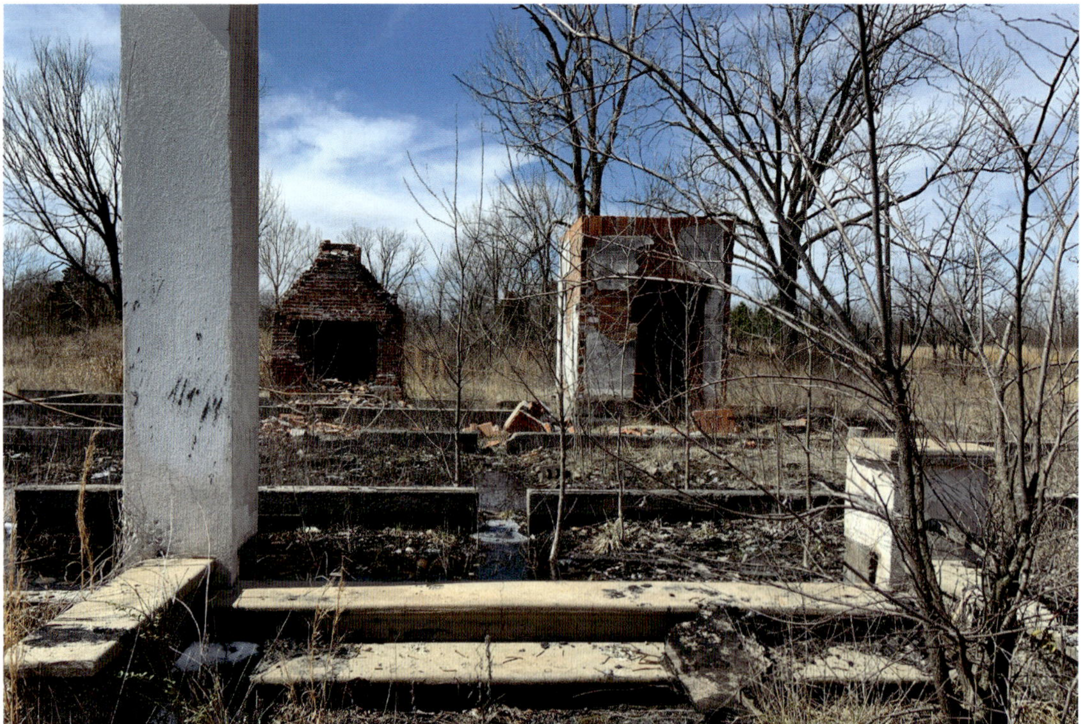

Front steps to the mining museum, March 2019.

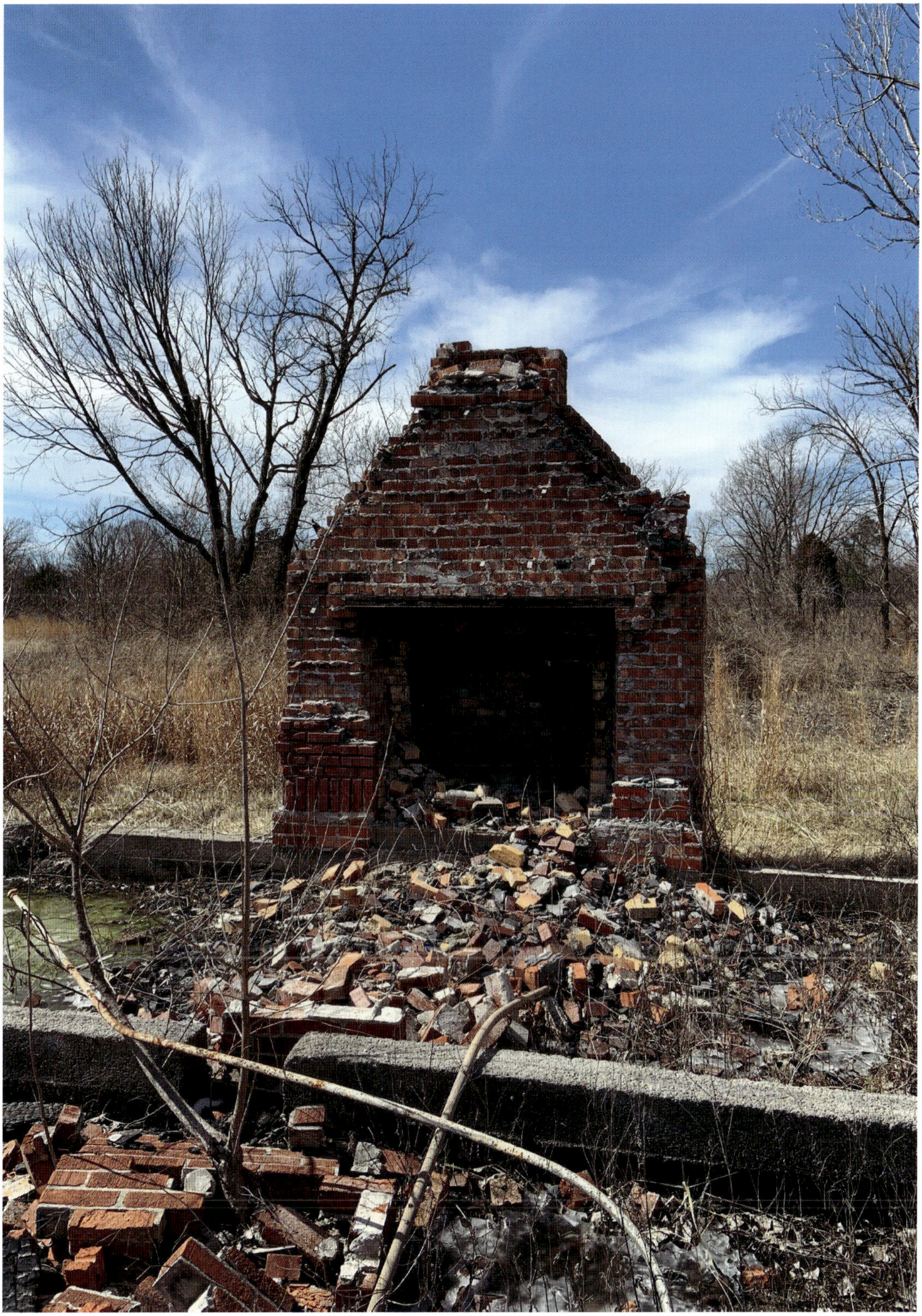

The fireplace that stood at the back of the mining museum, is only part of what it used to be, March 2019.

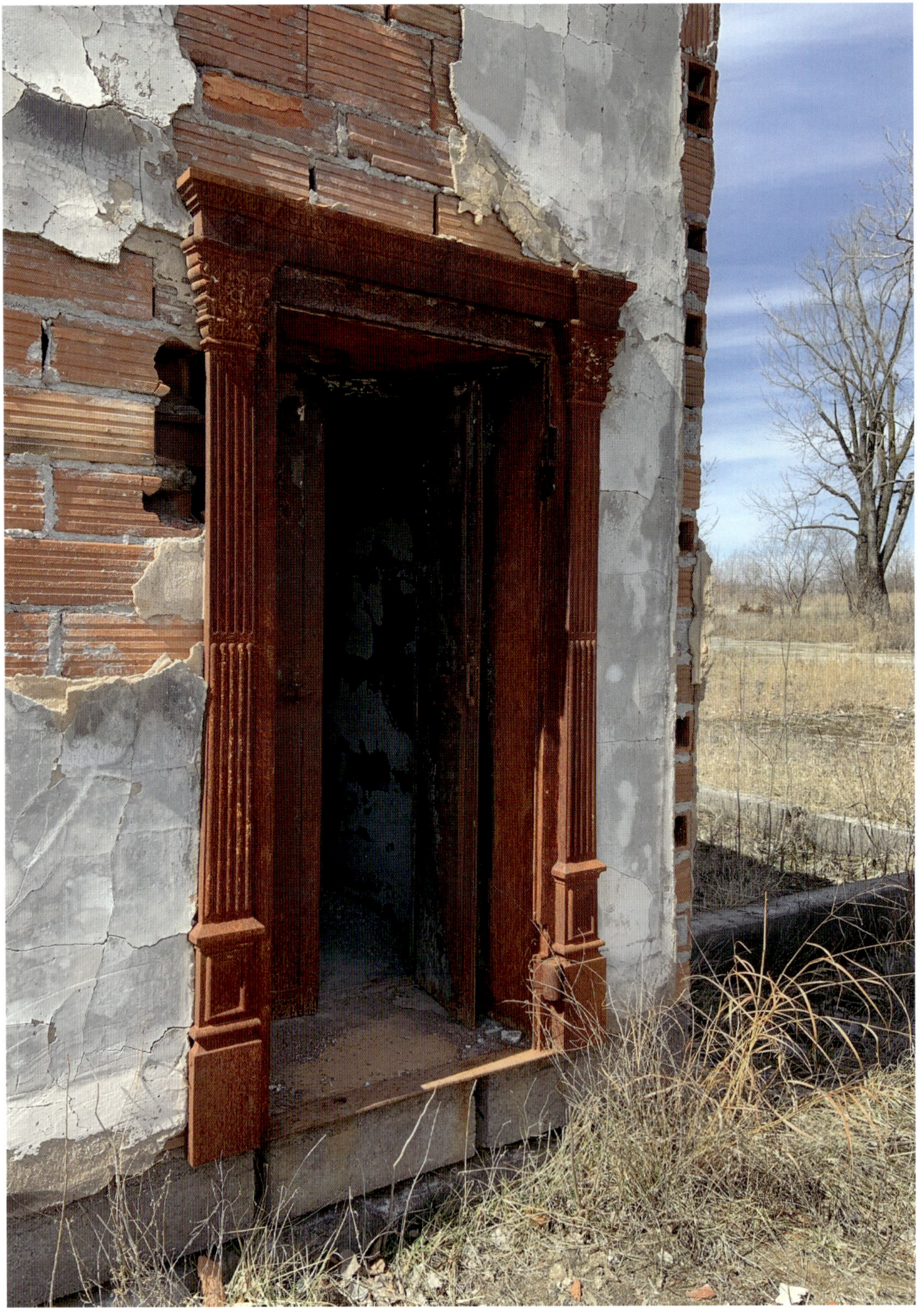

The mining museum's walk-in fireproof safe, March 2019.

As I walked around the complex, a police officer drove around more than once, watching what I was doing there. After seeing that I was just another photographer taking photos of the area, he did not seem all that concerned and drove away.

On the other side of the complex, I did notice that the building where Gary Linderman's pharmacy operated was still there, but the pharmacy closed when Gary unfortunately passed away from a "sudden illness" in 2015. He was only sixty years old. When the town did not even have a grocery store to speak of, Gary was there with his pharmacy to help those in need. The Town of Picher may still have residents; however, Gary kept his word to the town and the people. He did stay for the community, until he no longer could. Reading about him, I gathered that his death was a big loss to the remaining community that he cared so much for.

Just across the way from Linderman's pharmacy on Connell Avenue, the small strip of storefronts were now just empty spaces with only partial walls separating the former businesses. The houses behind the stores were still there as well. Surprisingly, not much had been touched in the houses. Furniture was still in the living room, personal belongings were scattered around, but this time around, the teddy bear that was in the back of the store had now made its way (50–60 yards) inside one of those house. There it was propped up under a window, as if it was waiting for me. I am sure that someone had simply taken it from its original location and left it in that house. I just found it odd that despite all the demolition, other onlookers, and workers for the cleanup efforts, this teddy bear still looked as it did the day I first saw it five years before.

The mobile home with the green kitchen and just frames for walls was still as I remembered it, just a little more worn from Midwestern weathering. I did not walk through the trailer because even though the frame may have proved sturdy, the floor was brittle and had multiple holes, making it unsafe to walk on.

Retracing my steps from my first visit, the gorilla statue was still on the corner in front of the city park, which this time was mowed, but was still fenced off. The gorilla appeared as if it got a fresh coat of paint and gloss not too long ago. I was happy to see the town mascot was still there but now freshened up from all the years of dust.

On the way to the school, I passed some of the same houses with the same signs of life as before. Although one of those homes, a mobile home by the school track was either purposely set or accidently caught fire in the middle of the home. The car and much of the homeowner's personal possessions were scattered everywhere as if the mobile home had exploded like a confetti popper. I could only speculate

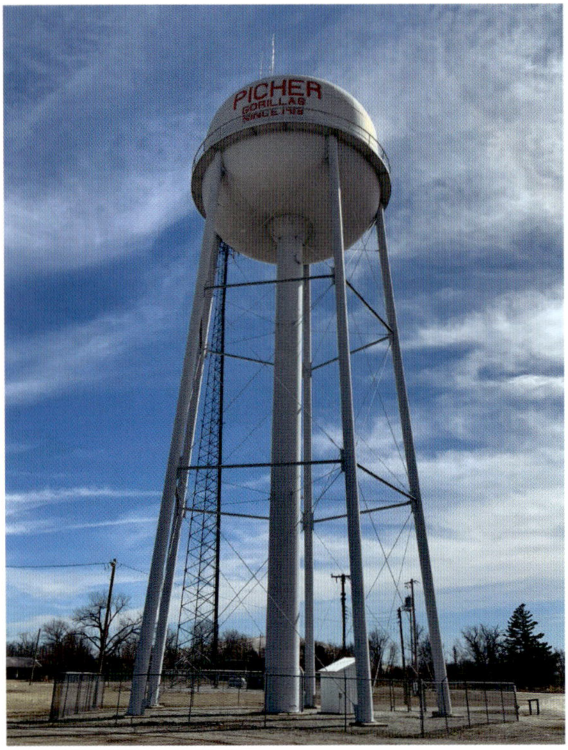

Left: The Picher water tower in March 2019.

Below: The ranch duplex complex in March 2019.

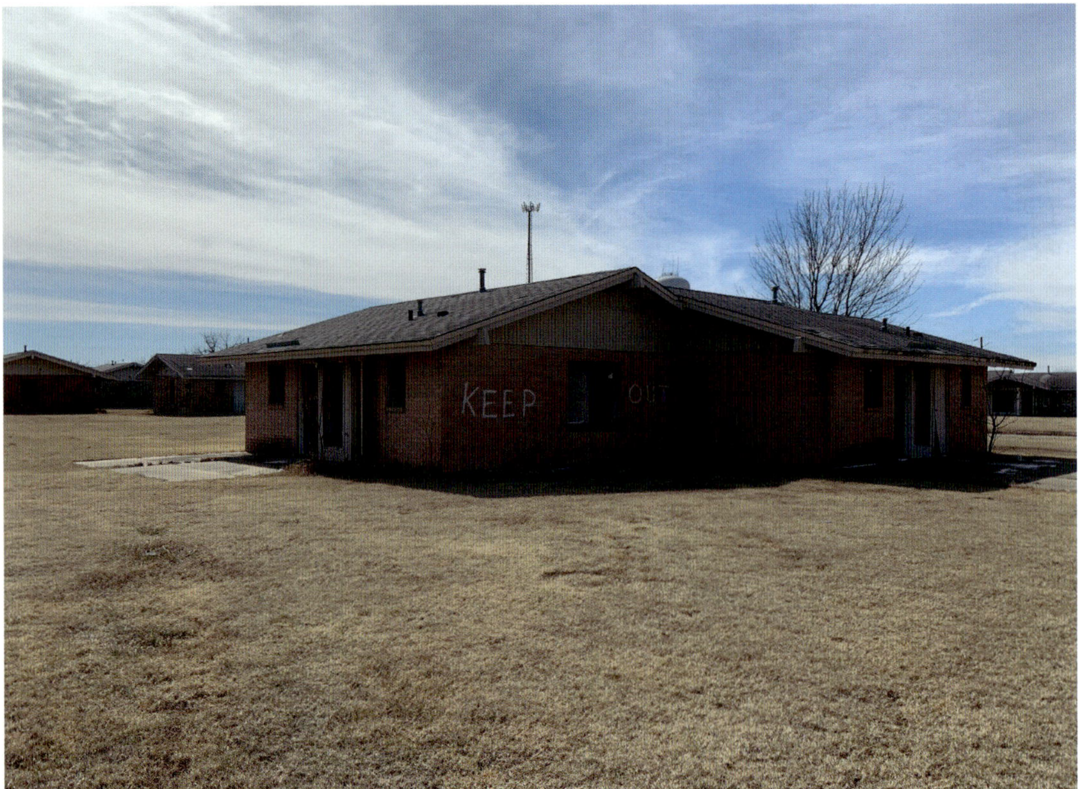

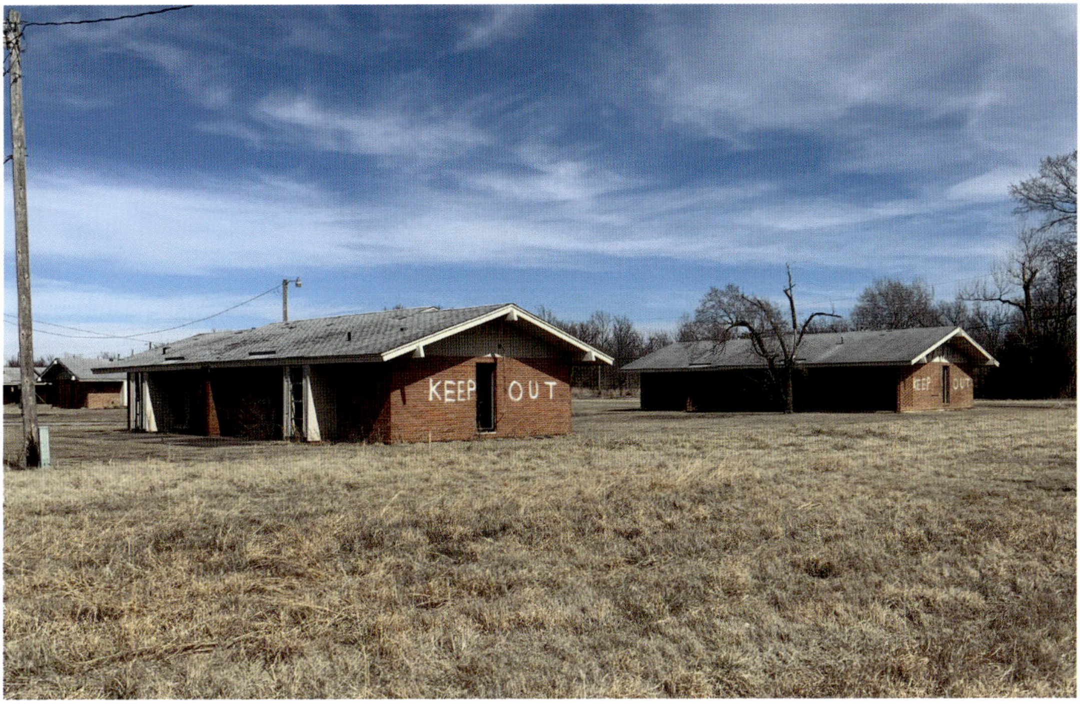

"KEEP OUT" still spray painted on the sides of the duplexes in March 2019.

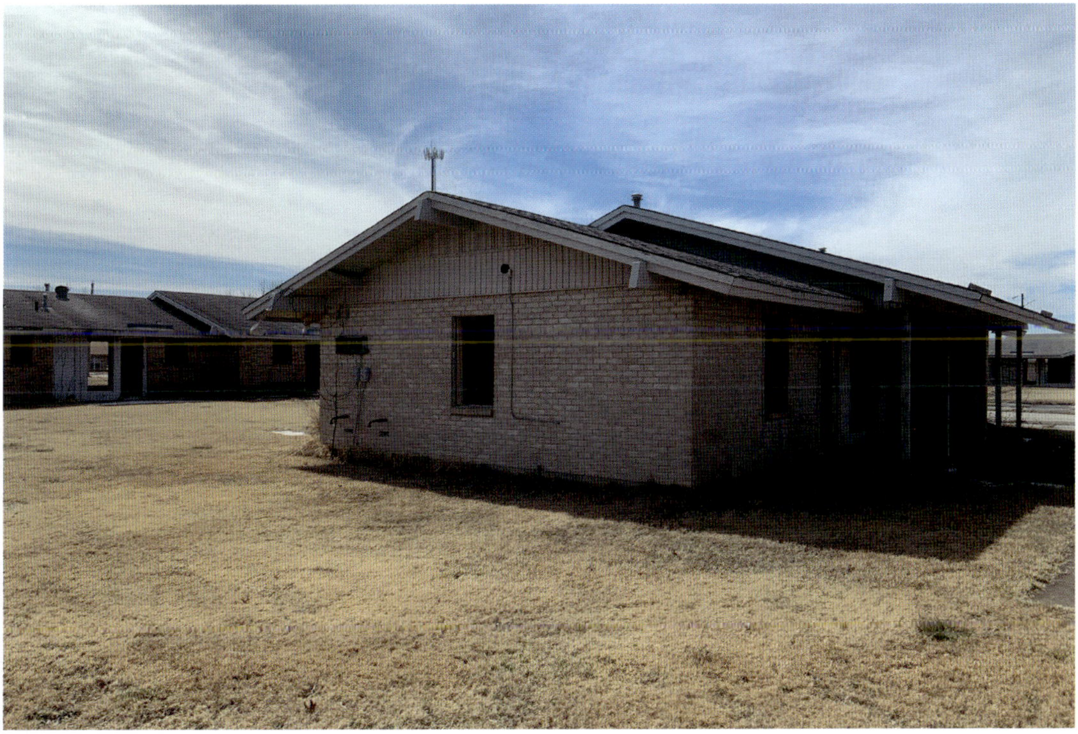

These are just a couple of duplexes in the complex on Devilliers Circle. The county sheriff's department has now moved into a couple of the duplexes in the same complex, March 2019.

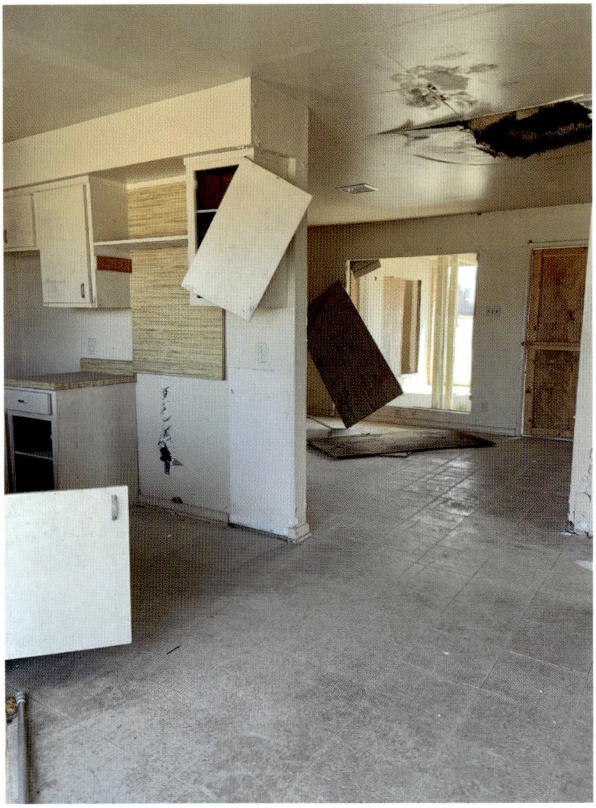

Left: Inside one of the duplexes, March 2019.

Below: Remains of the small strip of storefronts on Connell Avenue, March 2019.

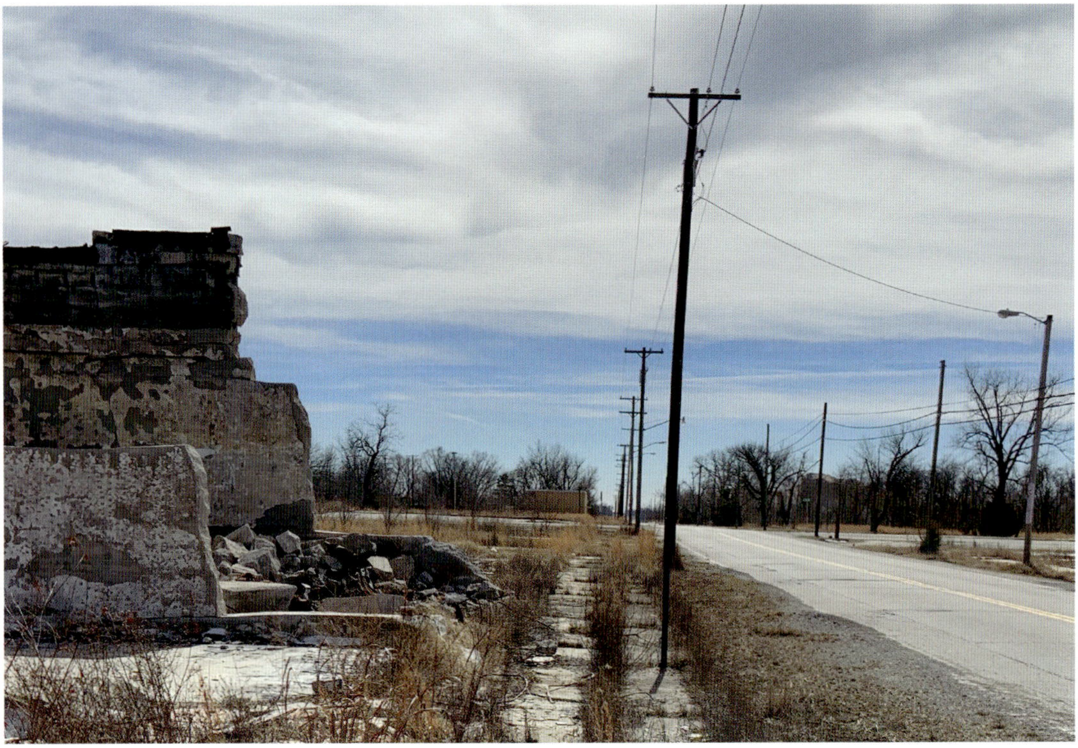

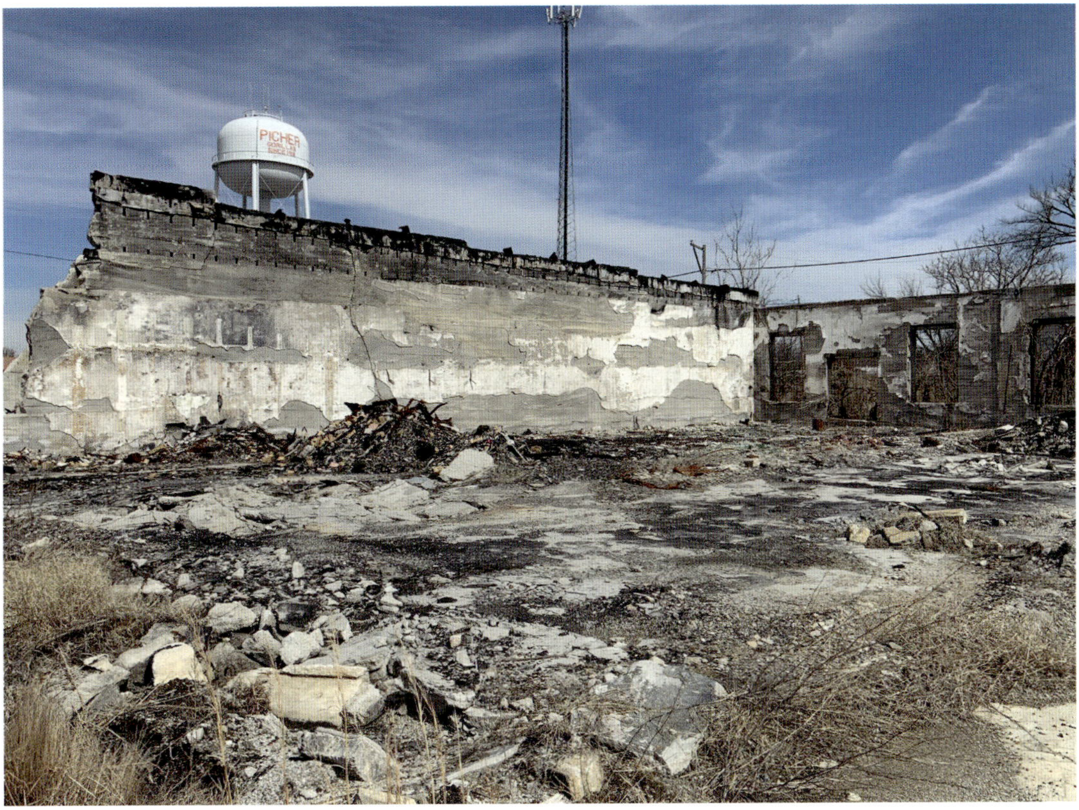

Above: Just a few feet down the sidewalk, this was once a business that operated on Connell Avenue.

Right: The last store in the row of shops—that was once beams and bare walls—is now only a partial building. This is also the same place where I found the teddy bear in 2014, March 2019.

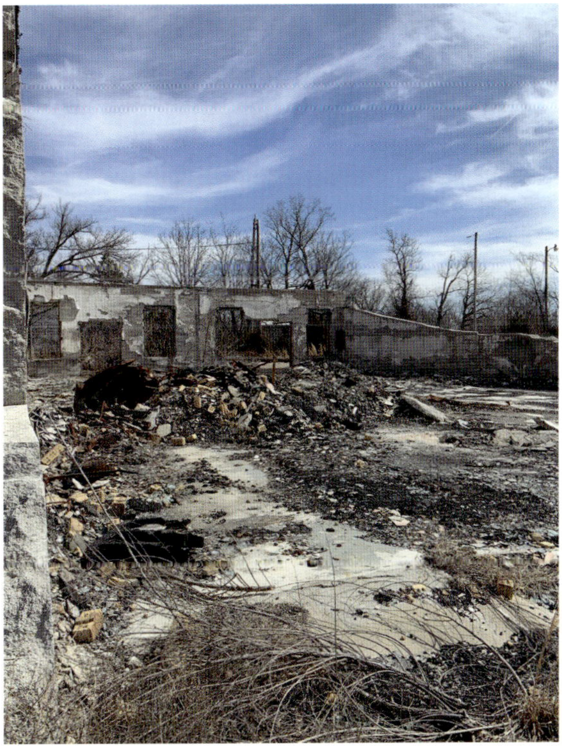

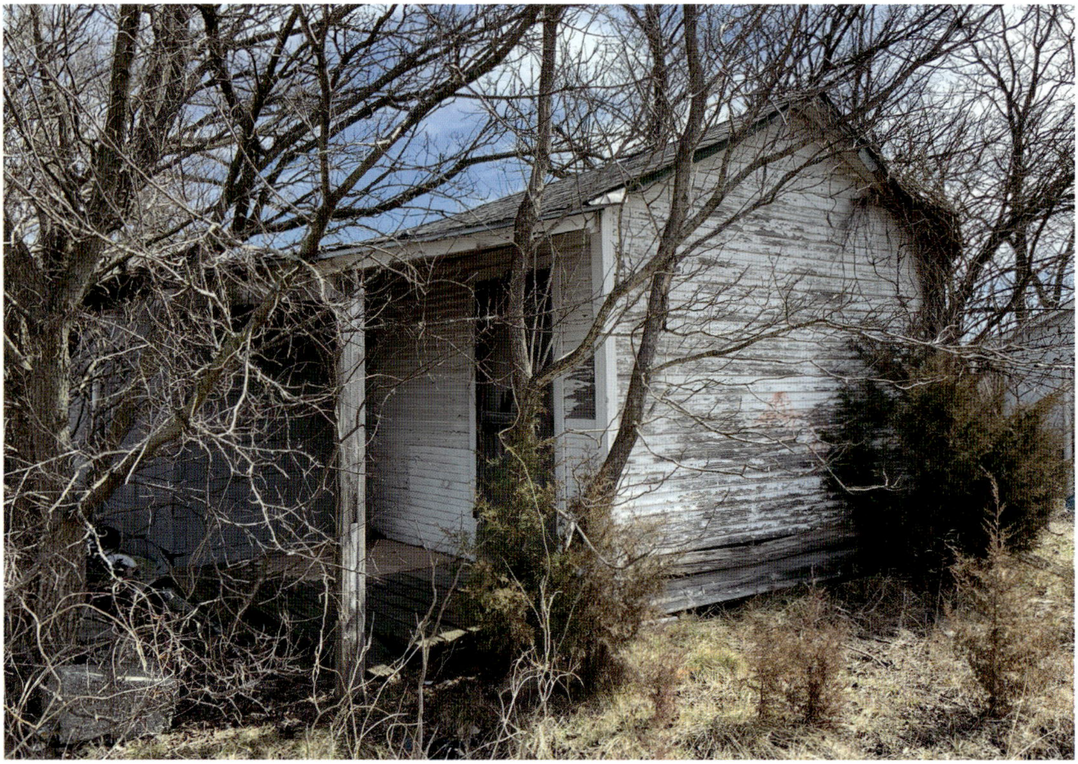

One of the houses behind the row of storefronts, March 2019.

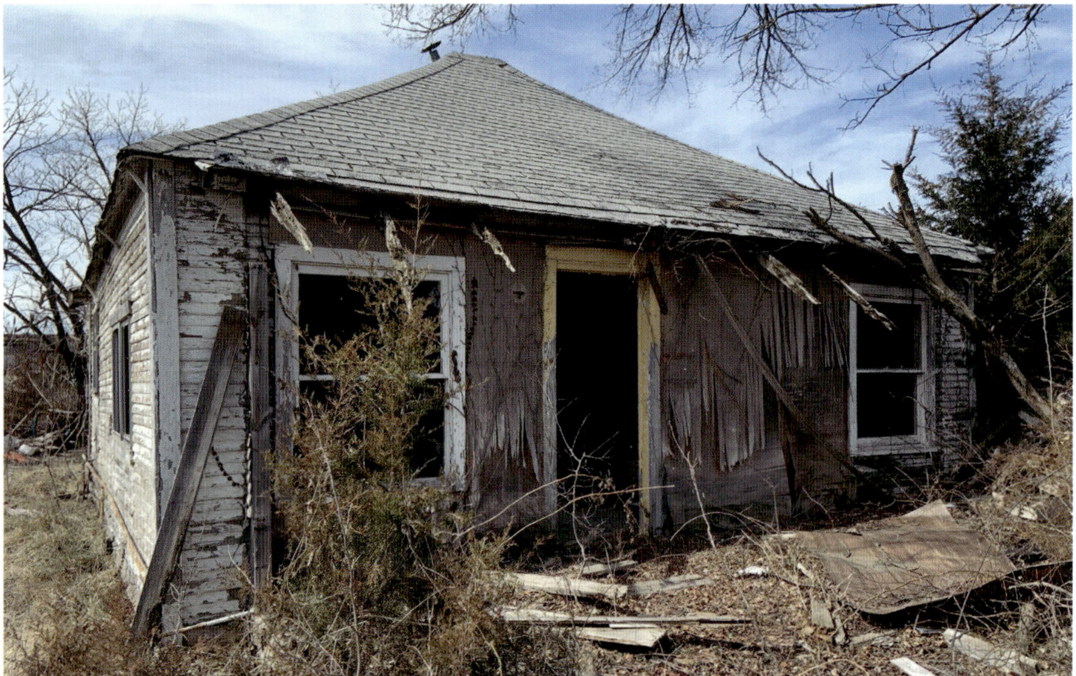

Another house behind the row of storefronts, March 2019.

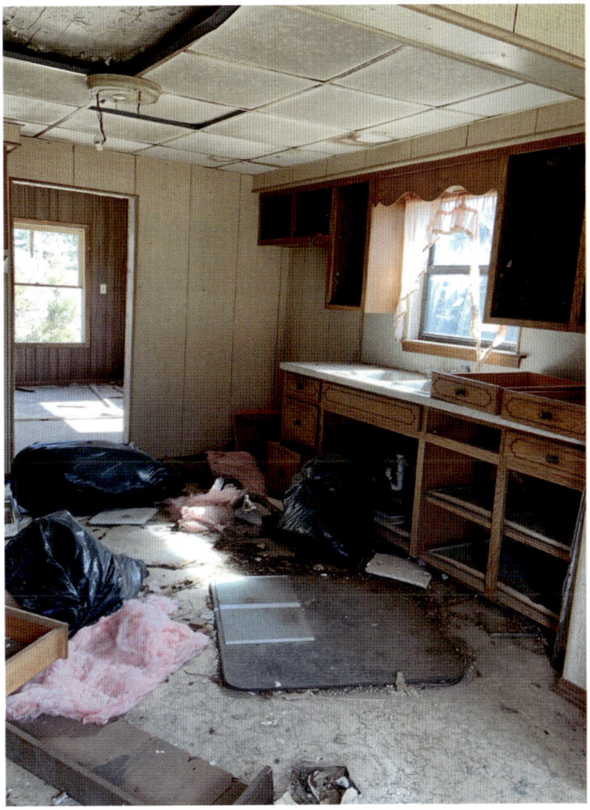

Right: Like the living room, the kitchen has not changed much since 2014, March 2019.

Below: Living room and same brown couch as before, March 2019.

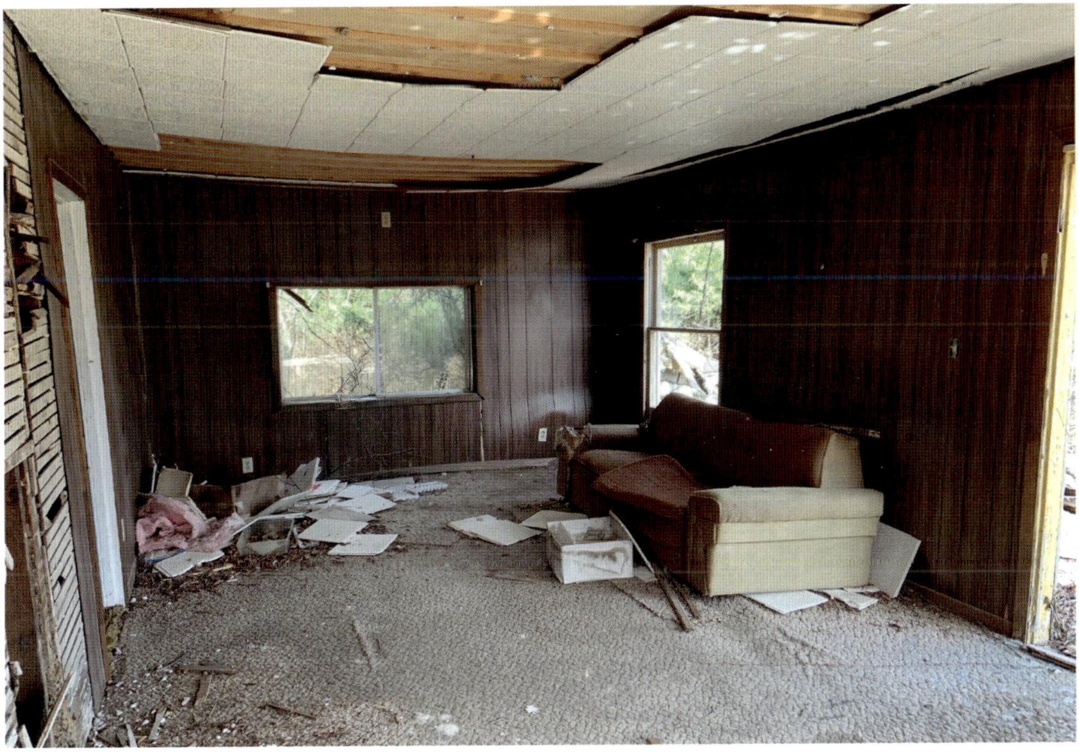

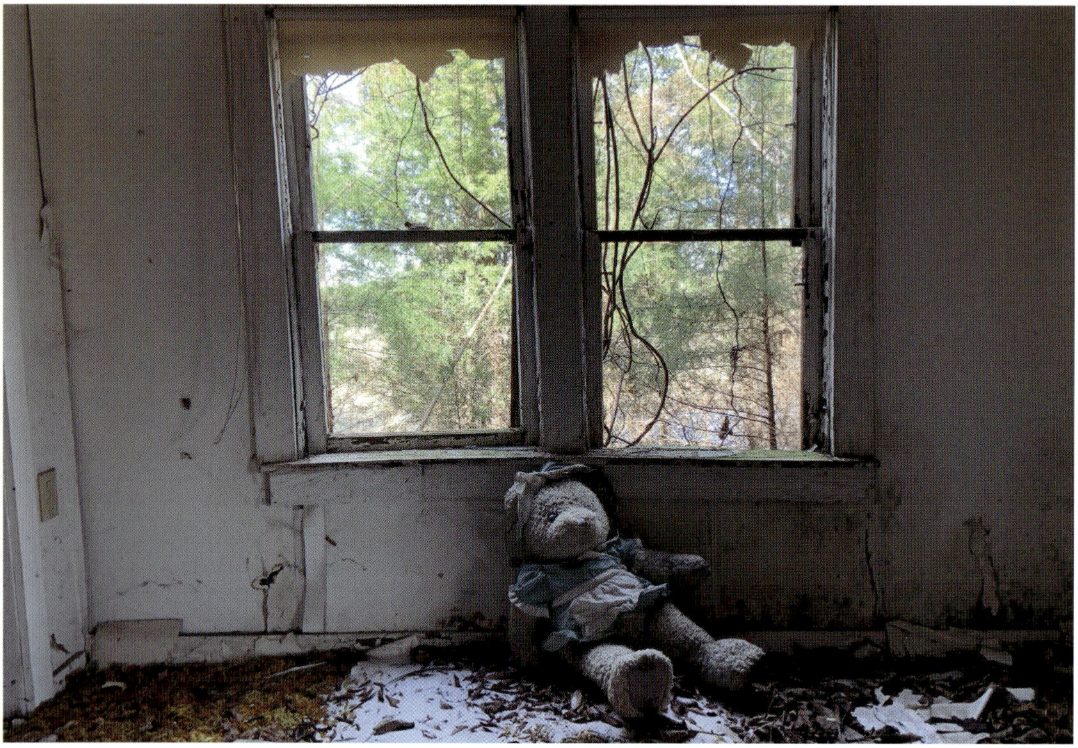

The teddy bear that once sat in the back of the last store has now made its way to the house behind the now crumbling stores, March 2019.

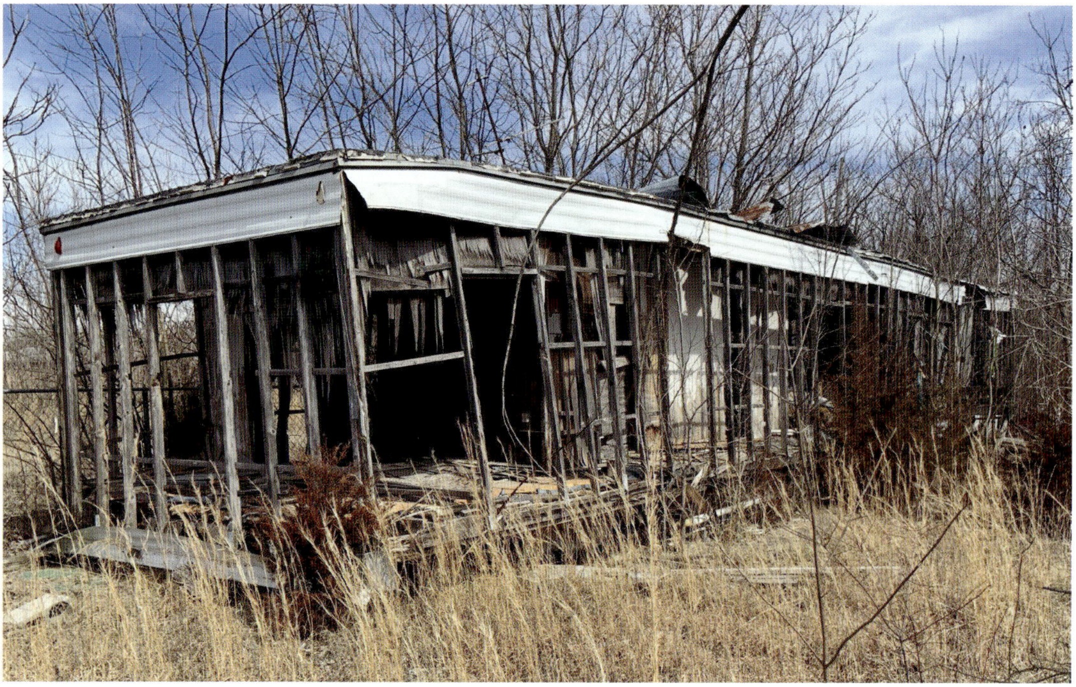

Despite not having any siding, the frame is surprisingly still holding this mobile home together, March 2019.

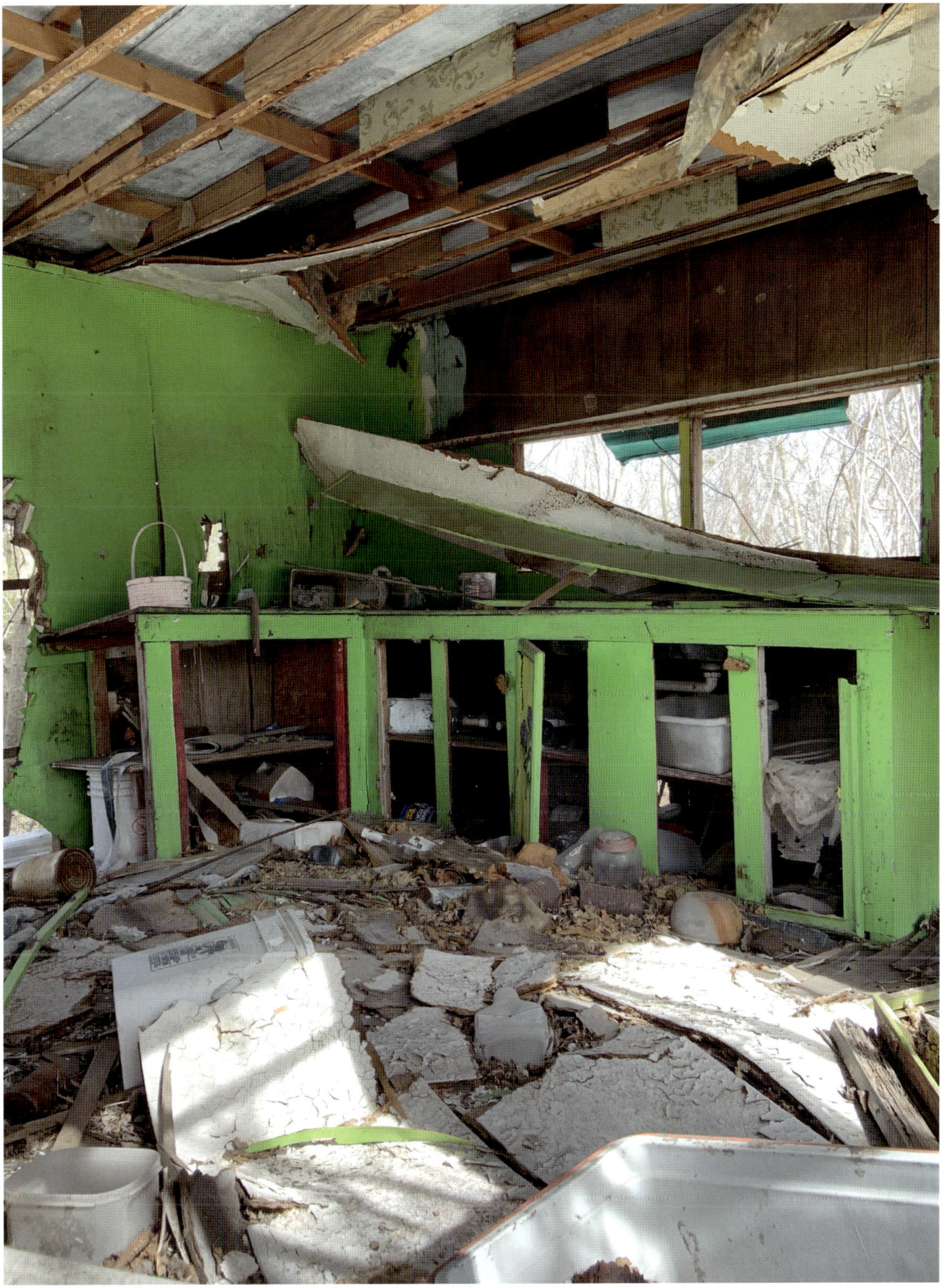

Bright green kitchen of that same mobile home. As well as the frame, the paint has also done a good job standing up to the elements, March 2019.

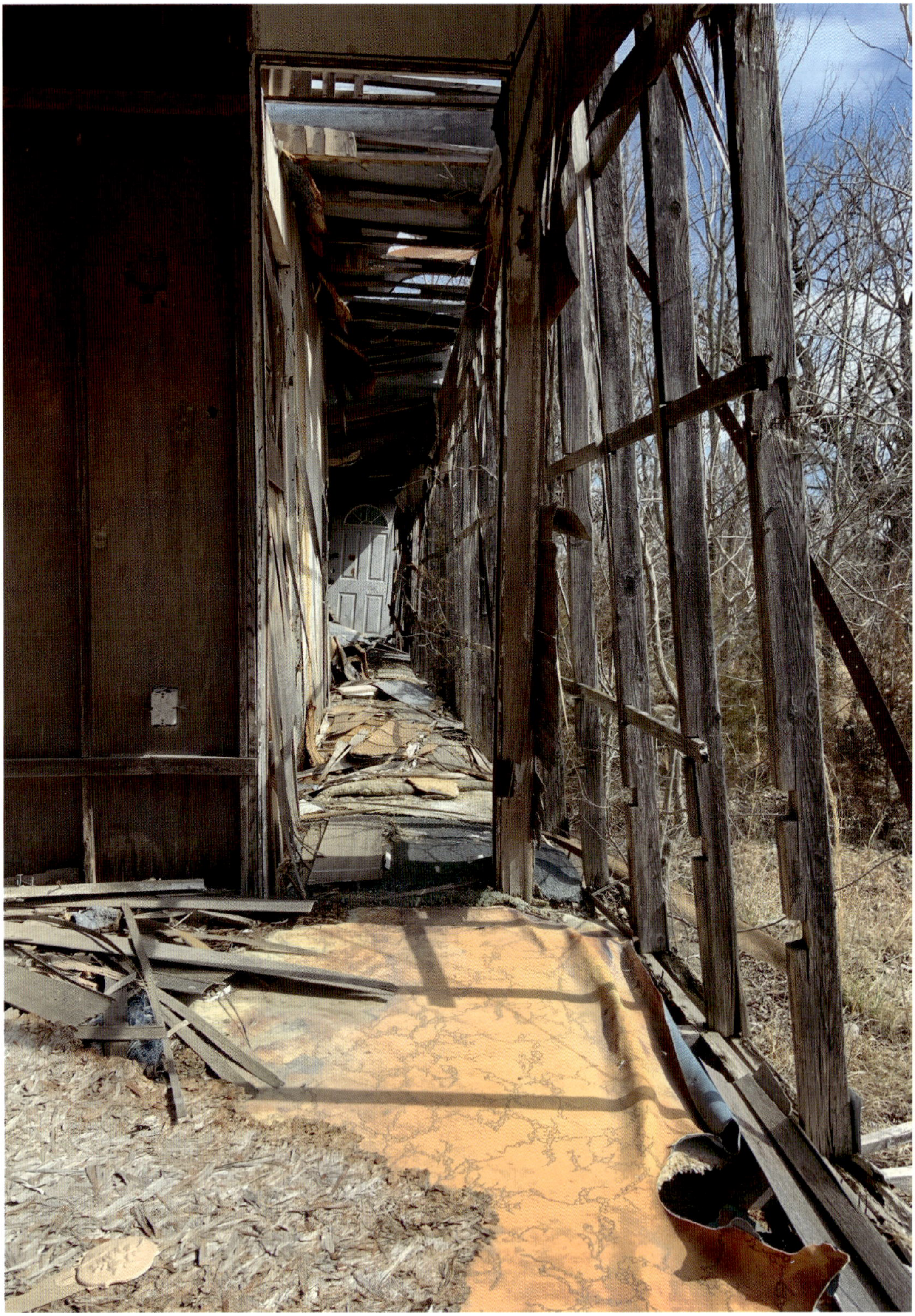

View down the hallway of the mobile home that has no siding, March 2019.

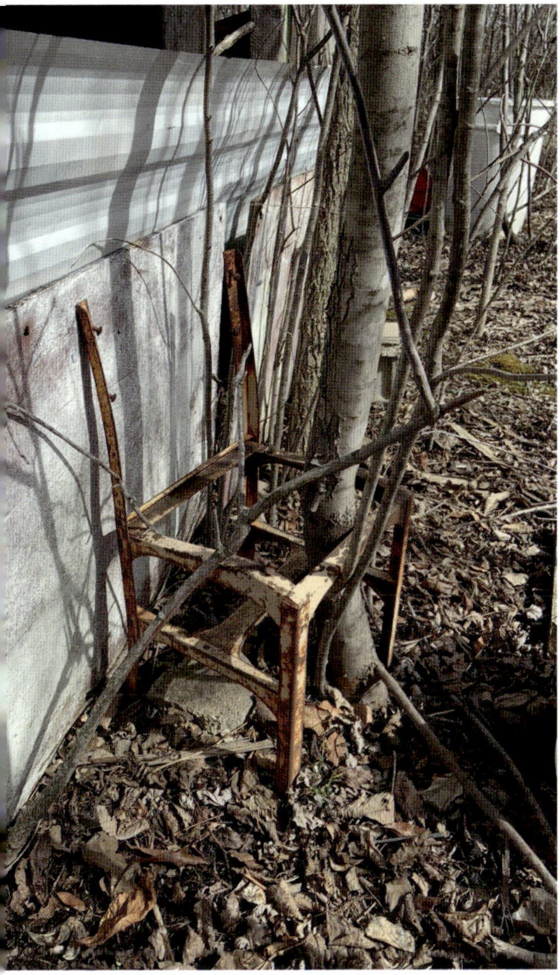

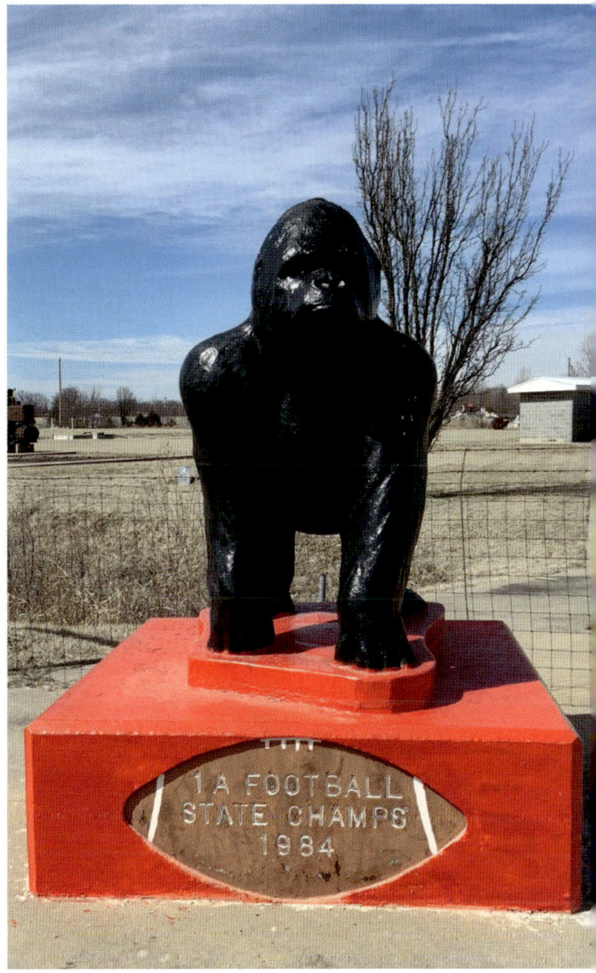

Above left: Tree growing through the rusted frame of a child sized school chair on the side of a mobile home, March 2019.

Above right: The Picher gorilla statue in March 2019. The park behind was mowed this time and the big rusty engine is still there.

if this was intentional and was it the same arsonist that had burned down other buildings around town. I did not ask the police nor did I find any articles in relation to this particular fire.

The school, track, and stadium was now completely surrounded by a reinforced 10-foot fence. The sheriff's station that was next door was now a construction or heavy equipment business. After asking permission from one of the supervisors, I was allowed to walk around the track and school to take as many photos as I wanted. Still neatly maintained the stadium and track looked the same. Honor roll names still displayed on the concession stand wall, the Coke scoreboard still stood at the end of the track, and the condition of the school still looked good.

While walking around the perimeter, there were signs posted everywhere that the school was now a training facility for county's law enforcement canine units. That did not stop me from trying to get in to take a look, especially since I did not get in the last time I was there. Entering the school would not be difficult either, since one of the side doors was left unlocked. I only went through part of the school to take photos for a few reasons: firstly, the lights were on, which usually means there's power, and power allows for surveillance or there could be people working there; secondly, the inside was in great condition, so there was not much to photograph; and last but not least, I am not trying to outrun or outsmart a police officer or his dog. I know my limitations and the consequences for evading the police. I checked out a couple classrooms. Some had desks, others were empty. The hallways were still painted with children's inspirational quotes and stick figure children all playing in a row. This school was probably in the best condition of all the schools I have explored. Being a small town, this school was also the smallest one I have explored. Going down one hallway, I had already seen and photographed half the school. Since I still had more of the town to explore, I left as quietly as I came before possibly getting into serious trouble.

After leaving the school, I went to the local public sports field that still also had their scoreboard and a small empty concession building. Like the city park and school track, the field was also mowed, but the baseball diamonds had faded all away and was just a grassy field by this time. I like to think that the remaining few residents take pride in their little piece of the world by working together as a team to take care of what was used up and left behind.

Then through a former residential area, there was a couple times when I thought I had encountered another abandoned home, but upon further inspection, there were indicators that people were living there. These homes were tucked away around a few turns here and there and beyond the overgrown plots of land. Driving by these homes and yards, my imagination thought that they looked like something straight

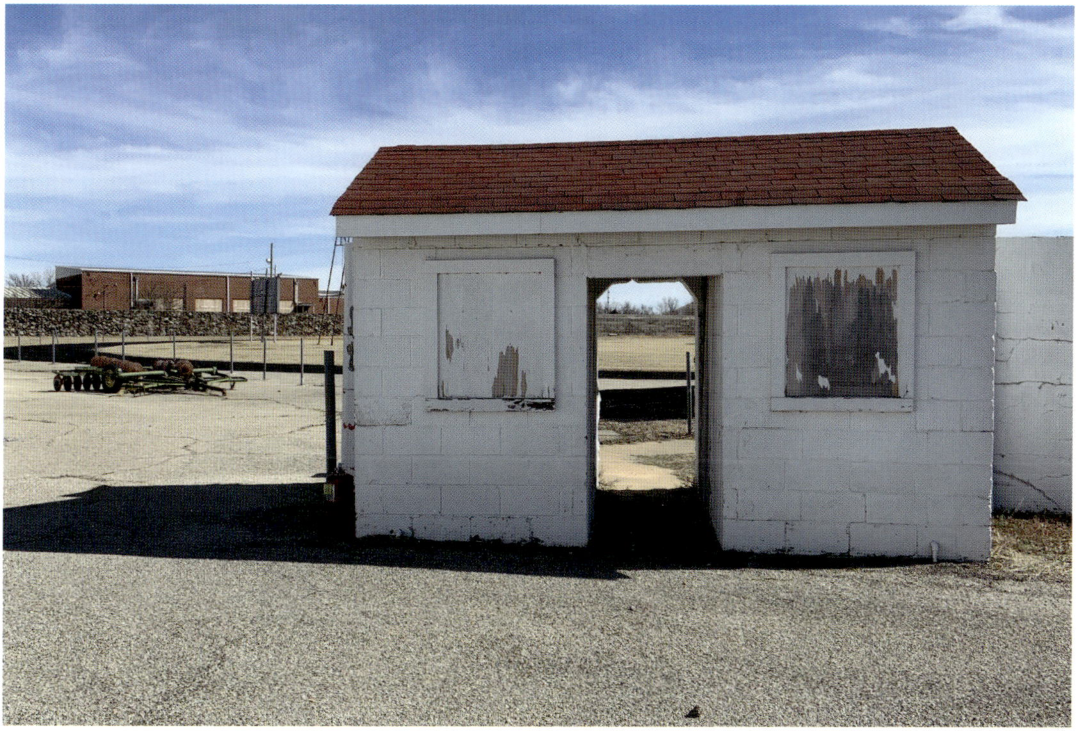

Entrance gate to the school track, March 2019.

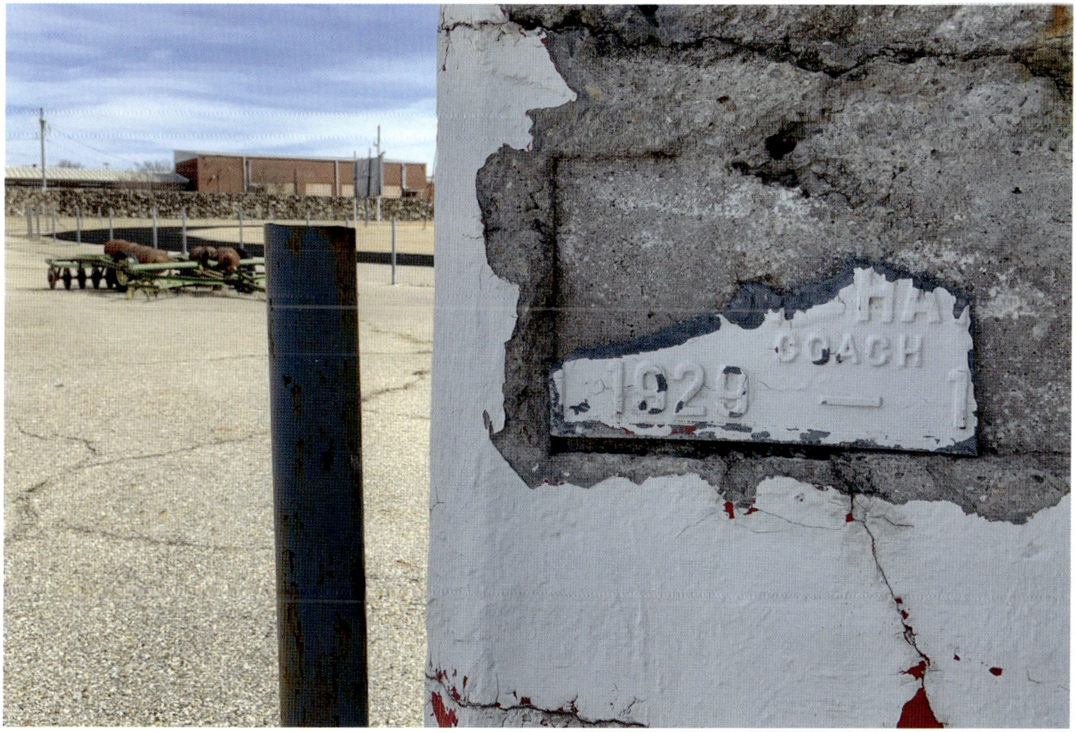

Broken plaque honoring one of the school's coaches, on the wall surrounding the track, March 2019.

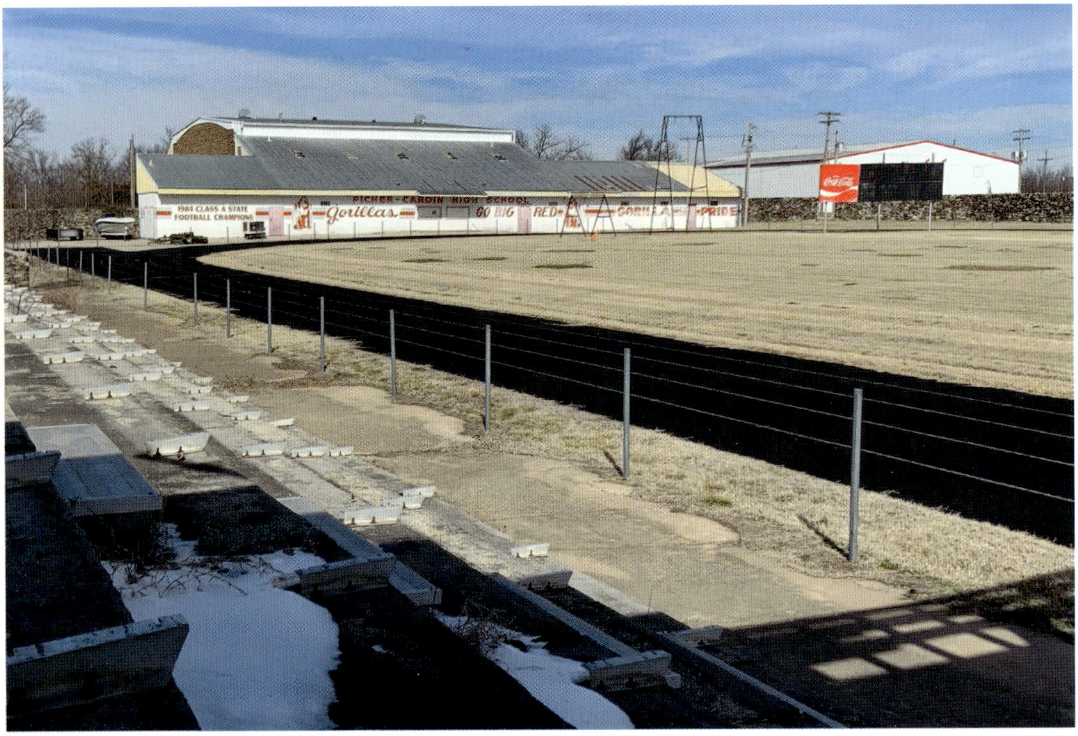

Minus the bleachers, view of the track, scoreboard, and concession stand from the bleachers, March 2019.

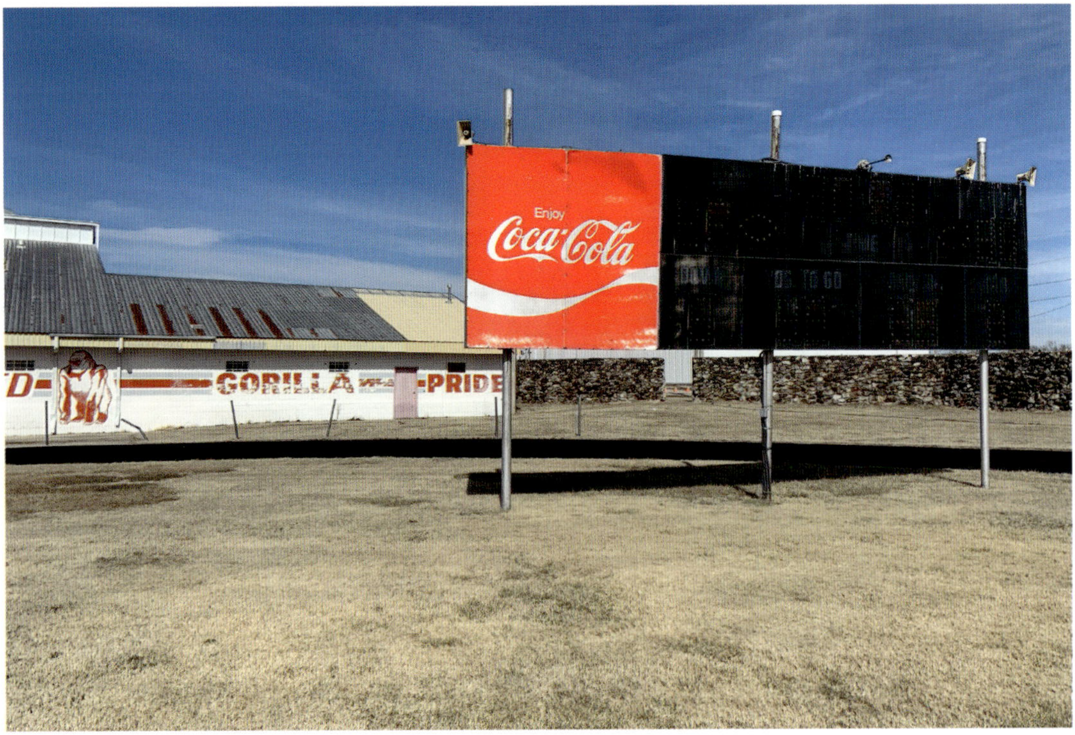

Slightly faded over time, the scoreboard's "time left" and "yards to go" is still visible enough to read, March 2019.

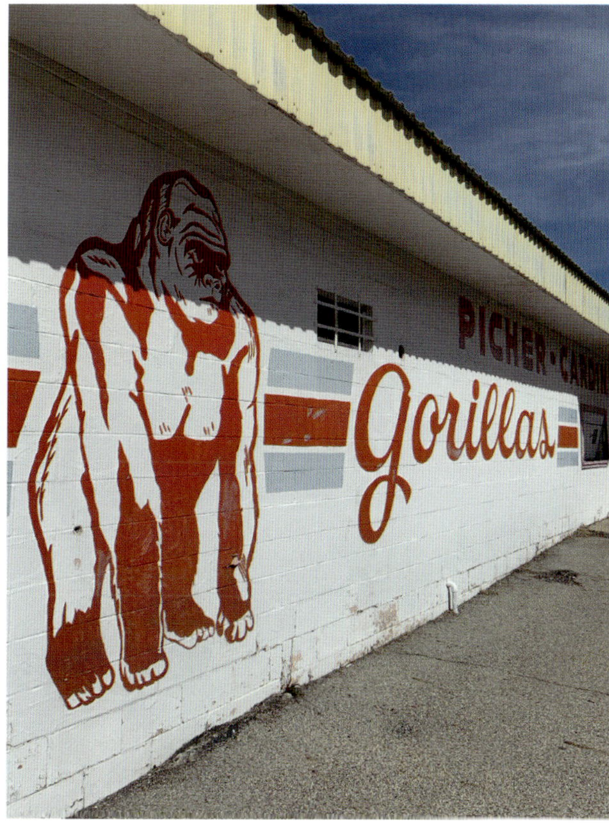

Right: Picher-Cardin Gorillas mural on the wall of the fieldhouse/concession stand building, March 2019.

Below: Front view of the fieldhouse/concession stand building, March 2019.

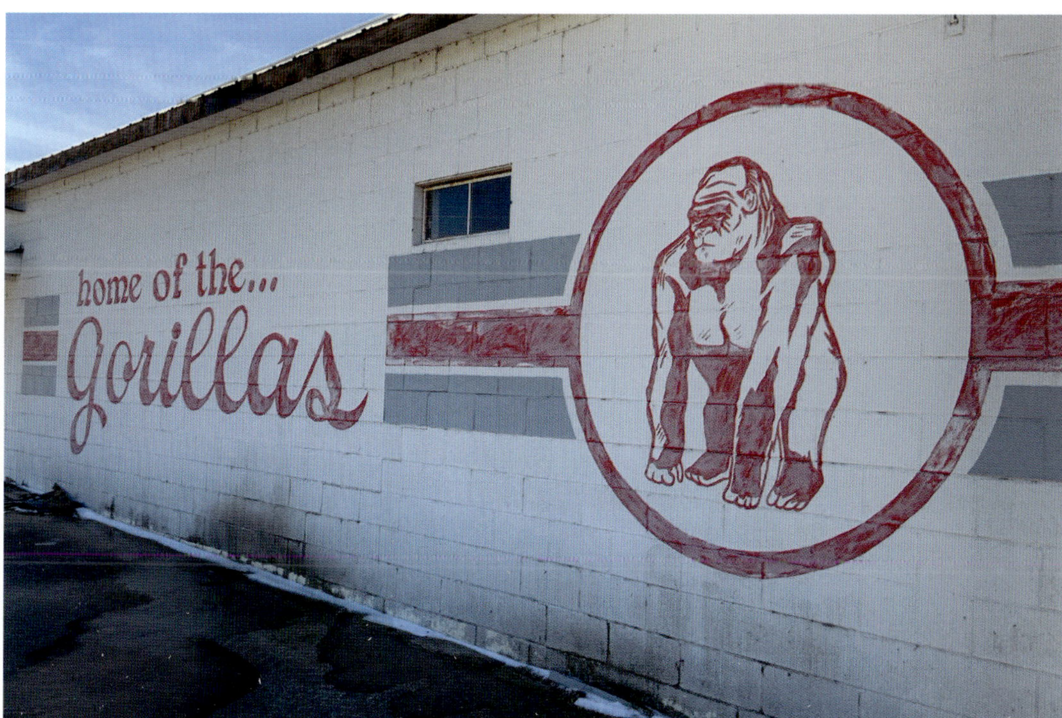

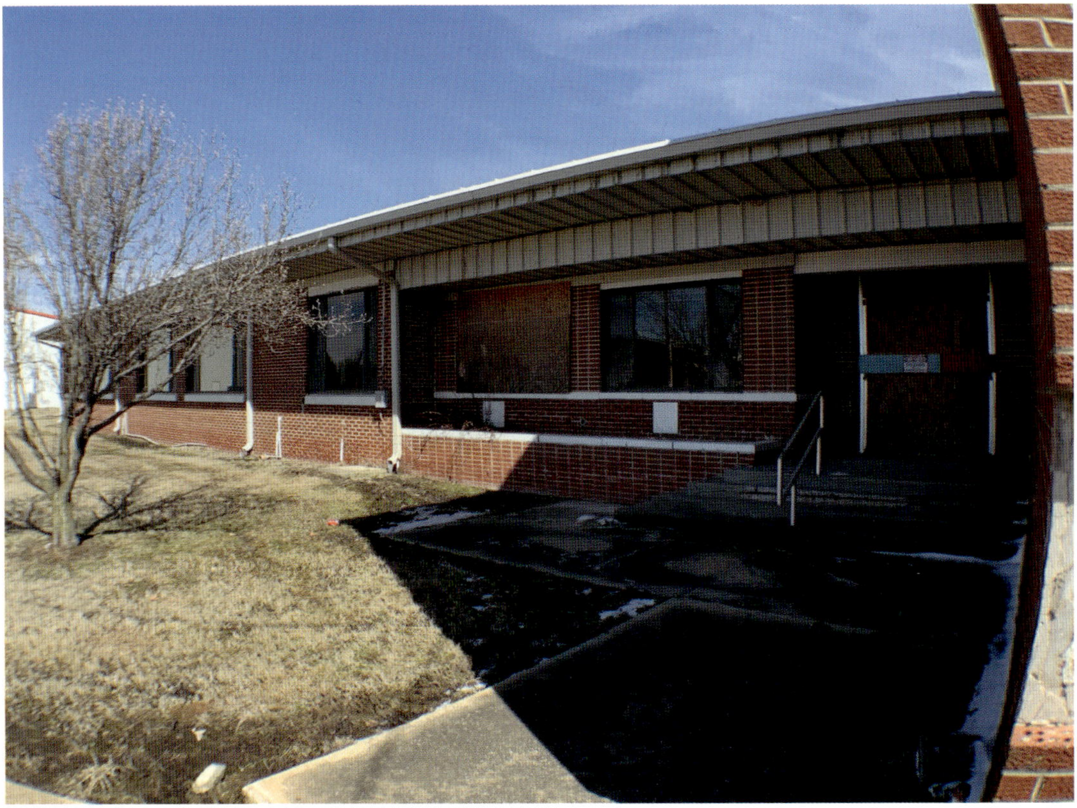

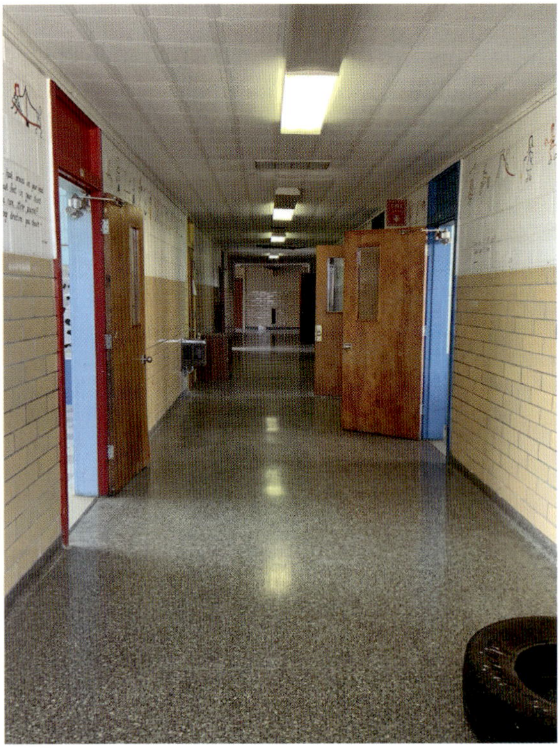

Above: Front entrance to the school. Currently being used for police training, March 2019.

Left: View down one hallway of the school. One of the nicest schools I have had the privilege of exploring, March 2019.

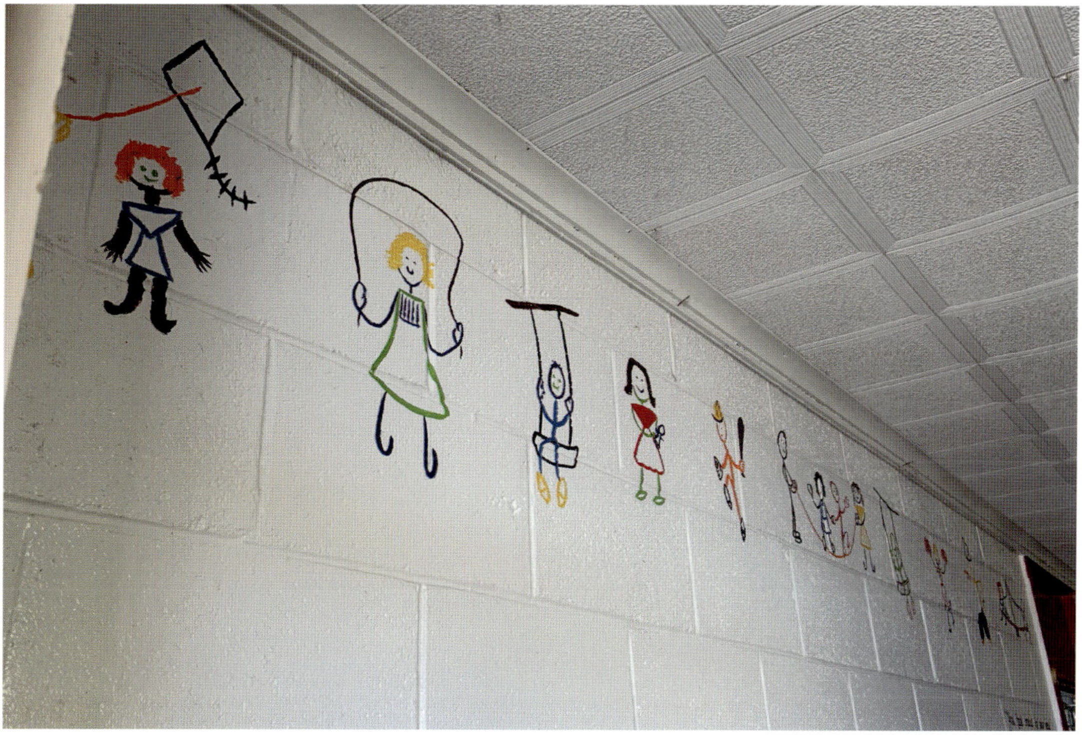

Stick figure children playing are painted down the whole hallway, March 2019.

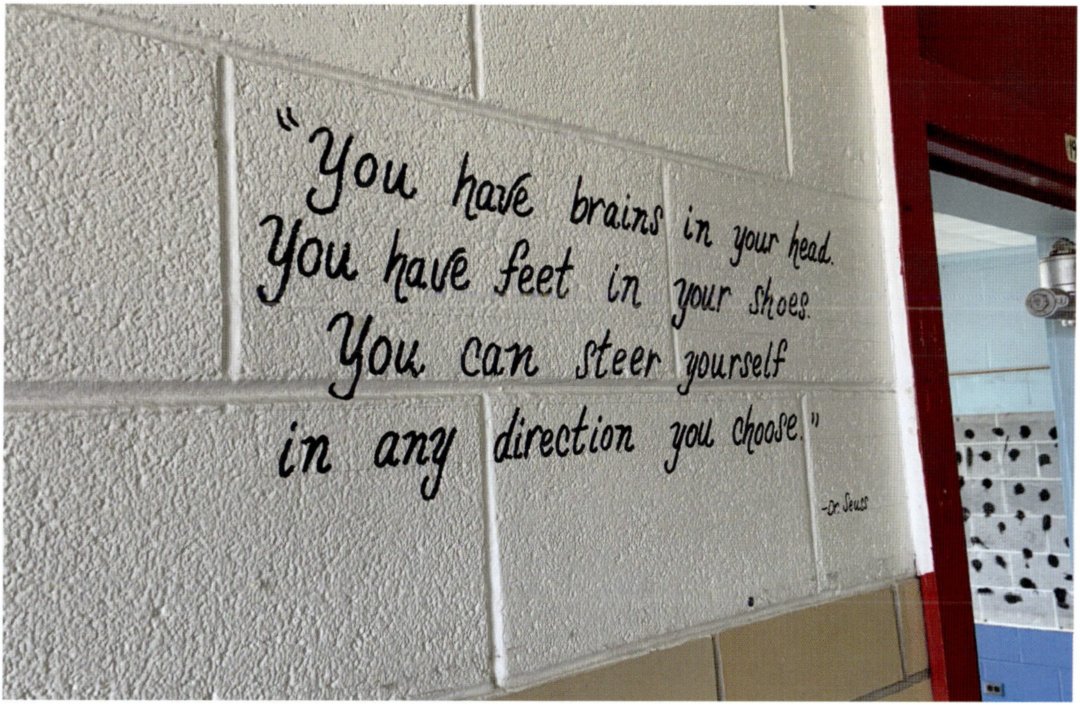

Inspirational quotes are still painted by the doors of each classroom. This quote from Dr. Seuss reminds children that their future is full of potential, March 2019.

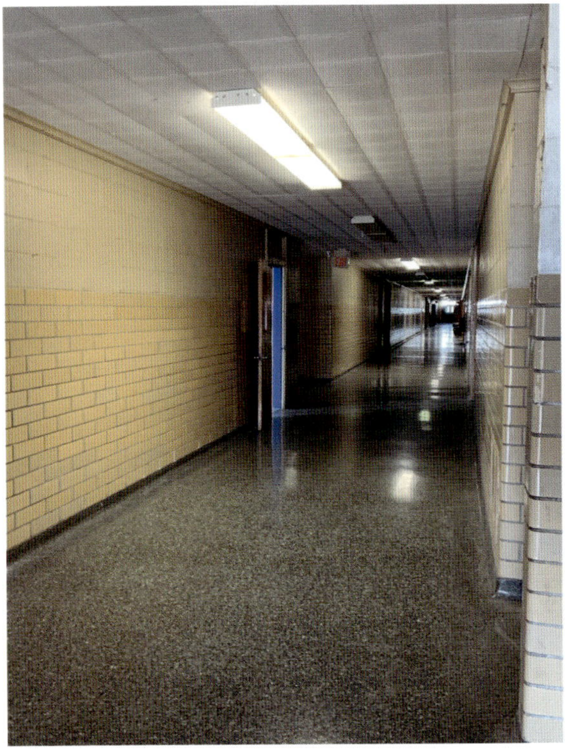

Left: View down the main hallway of the school, March 2019.

Below: Classroom full of desks. Through the windows you can see another chat pile that surrounds the area, March 2019.

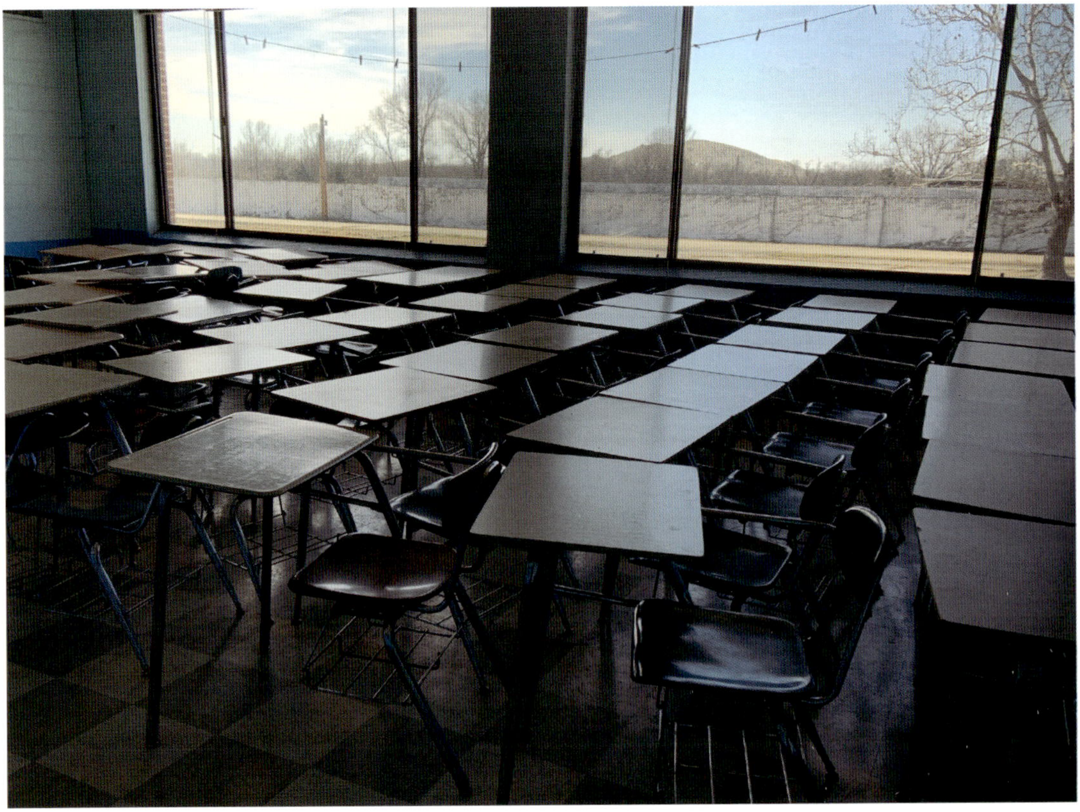

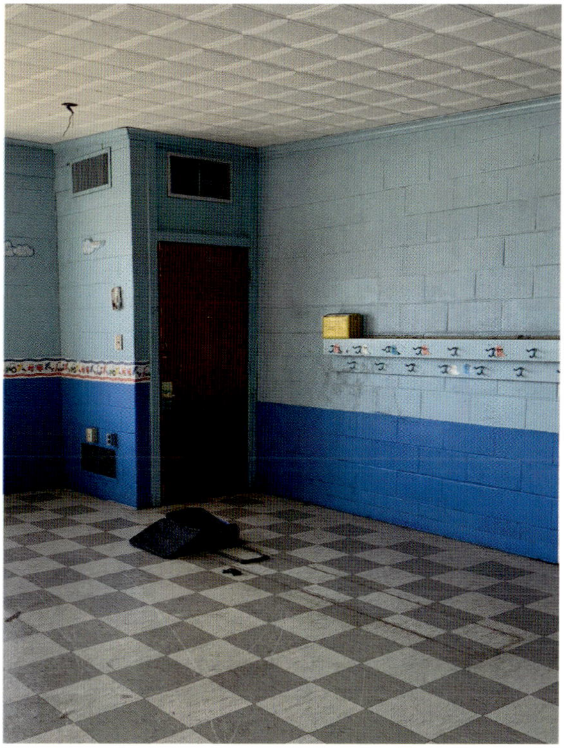

Right: Where children once learned how to read and write is now an empty classroom, March 2019.

Below: Walking up to the back of the school from the track, March 2019.

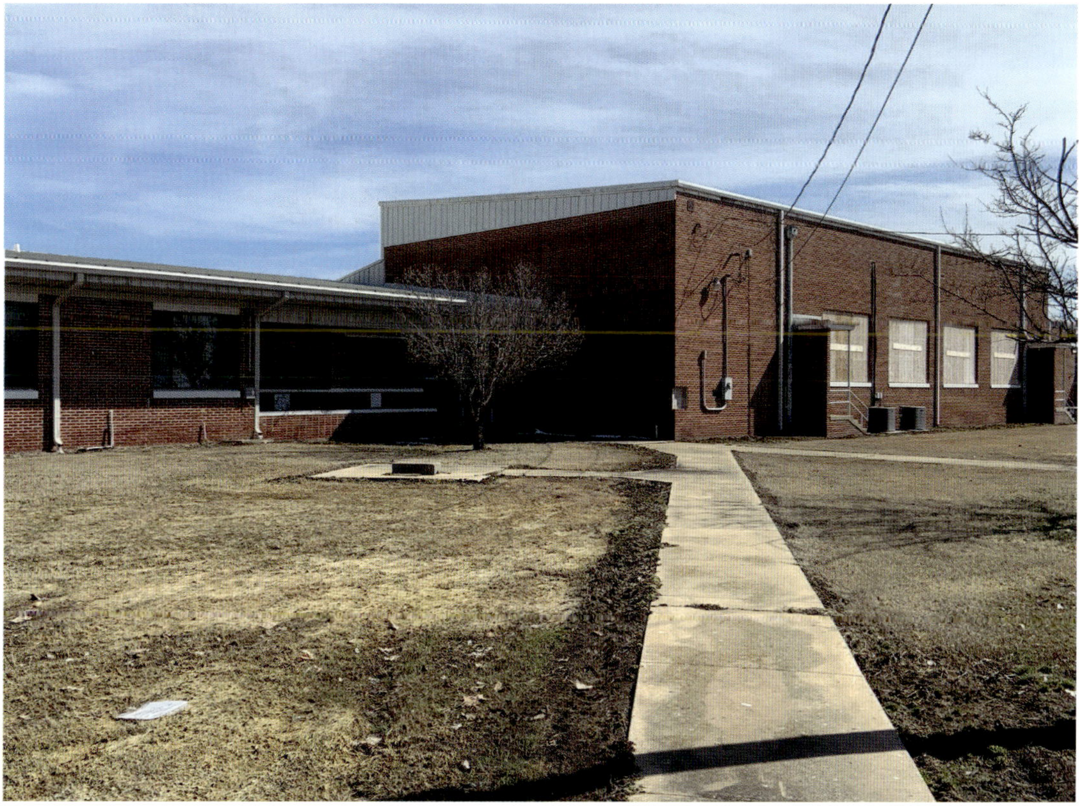

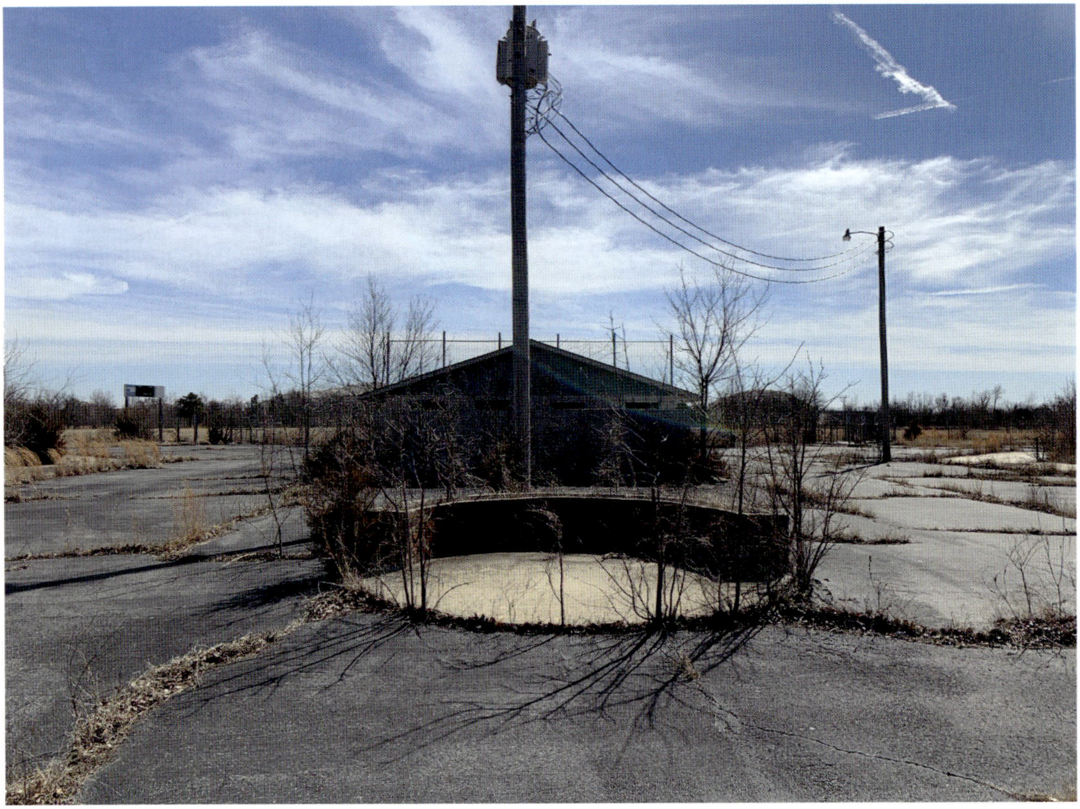

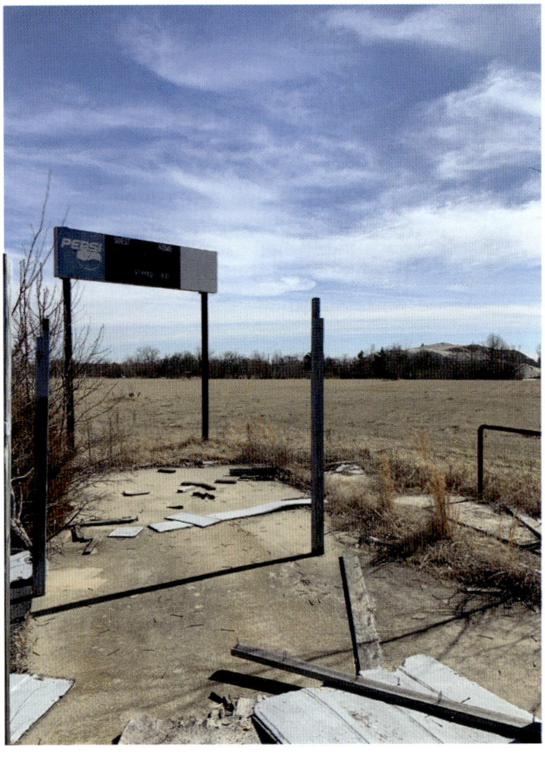

Above: Once a place where the people of Picher gathered to play baseball, now the diamonds are faded away and there are no bases left to run, March 2019.

Left: Home and Guest has not faded from the scoreboard that still stands right before entering the field, March 2019.

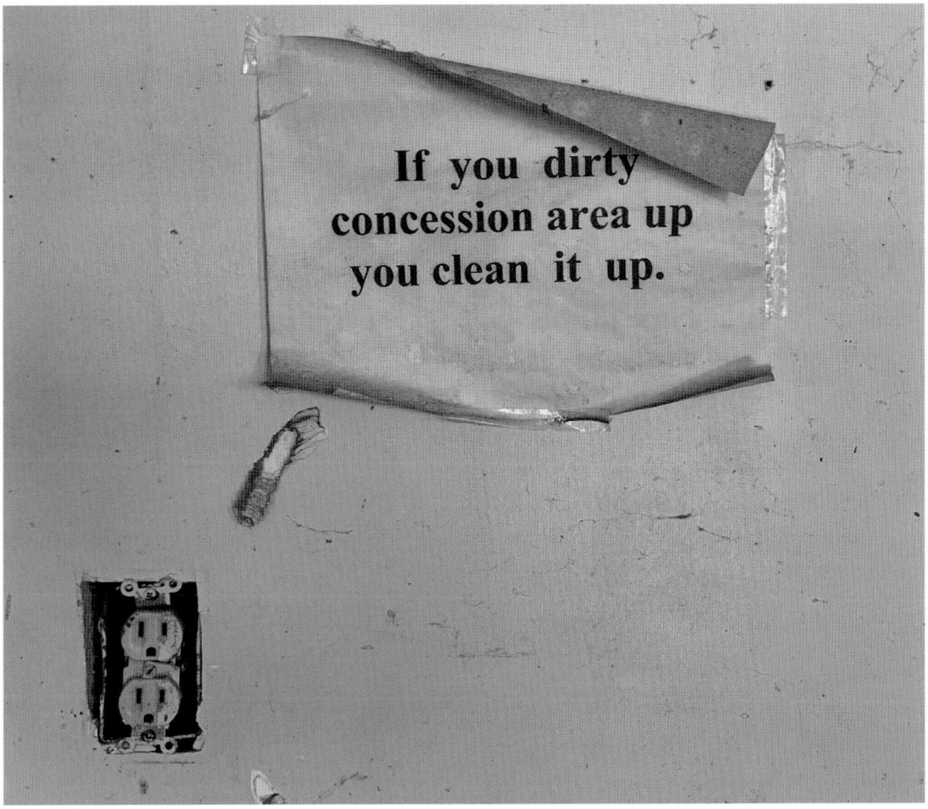
If you dirty
concession area up
you clean it up.

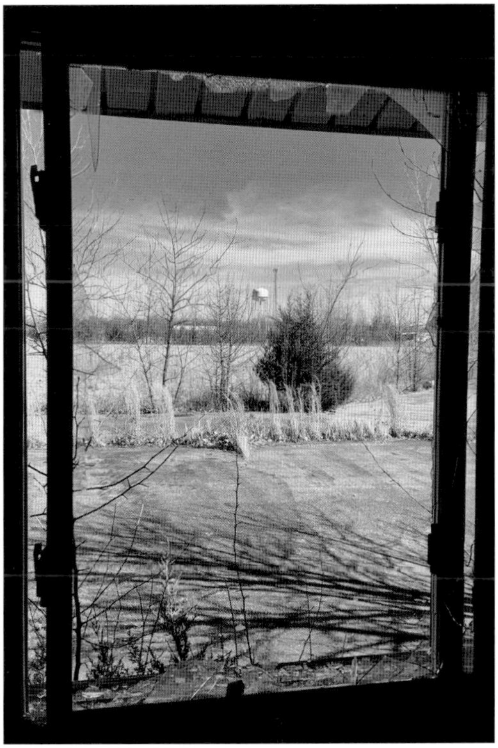

Above: The sign for concession stand employees still hangs on the wall, March 2019.

Right: View of the Picher water tower through broken window of the ball park's concession stand, March 2019.

out of a horror movie. But when I drove by, those who were out front were very cordial by waving and smiling. Also tucked away in the same back wooded area was a church. On the corner of North Treece Street and "B" Street, what I thought was one of the bigger homes in town was actually the Full Gospel Revival Church. I did not even get through the front door before I encountered an old, faded green piano covered with a green and orange shag carpet. Sounding horribly out of tune like demented circus music, the piano still played. Entering into the church, there was boxes of rusted can goods, old VHS tapes, and a couple creepy baby dolls all over the big one-room church. The walls were starting to mold and part of the ceiling was gone due to years of water damage. Once a place of worship, is now beginning to fall in on itself.

Out the back door of the church, there was a small gold and cream colored vintage camper. The inside wood paneling was surprisingly in good condition despite the doors and windows being left open. What used to be yellow curtains are now just torn and tattered shreds hanging from a curtain rod. The owner's contents, from an old record player to more canned goods, were thrown about everywhere inside and out. The randomness of possessions laying all over the ground, not just at this home, but many of the homes left standing in Picher, ranged from a bunch of kids toys and baby dolls to kitchen utensils.

After finding that unexpected church and vintage camper, I was still trying to locate that bigger church I photographed on my first visit. I was really hoping that it was still in the same condition as it was before. I drove around in circles for a few minutes looking for the Christian church. Unable to remember exactly where it was, I decided to ask the local police. The very nice police officer informed me that it was burned down in 2017 and that the arsonist was never apprehended. I wish I had gotten more photos the first time, because there was no second chance to get those now.

Almost back to the main road, there was a long mobile home-type structure with no signs indicating what it used to be, except for the word "Picher" painted on the front. With a little more digging, I found it used to be the Picher Auction house. That would explain why I found another piano left behind inside. Like the first piano, this one was also in terrible condition. The building itself was heavily damaged and all the walls were either covered in graffiti or the sheetrock had been punched through. Having been through a lot of the buildings in town at this point in the day, this building had borne the brunt of destructive vandals. Other places had obviously been gone through and things moved around; however, there was no graffiti and deliberate damage.

There was just a few more houses to check out before leaving town. A couple of these were in too bad shape to safely go inside, but it was not hard to take interior photos

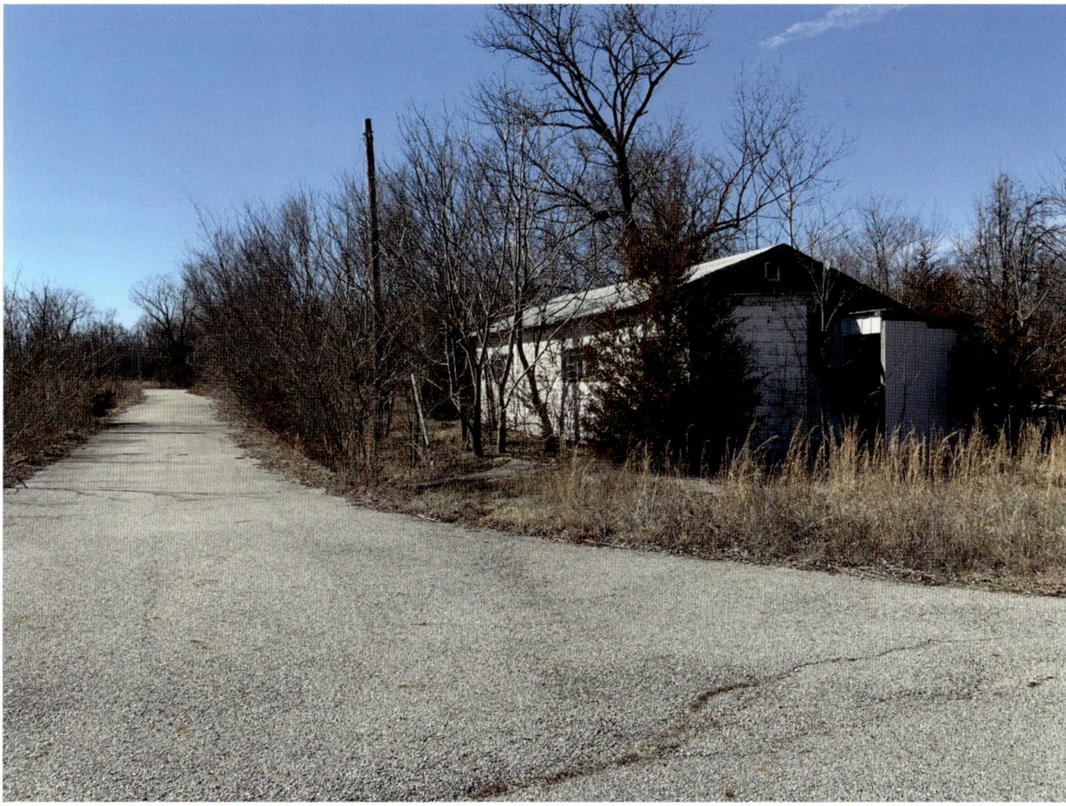

Above: Street view of the Full Gospel Revival Church, March 2019.

Right: Entrance to the Full Gospel Revival Church, March 2019.

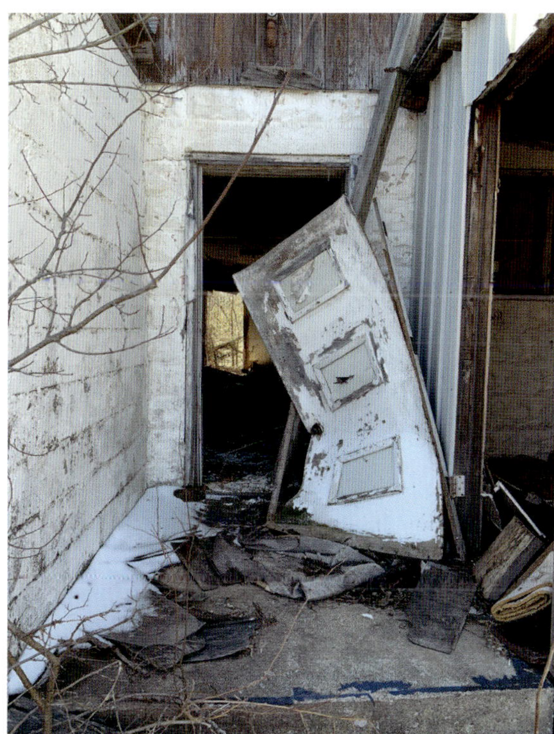

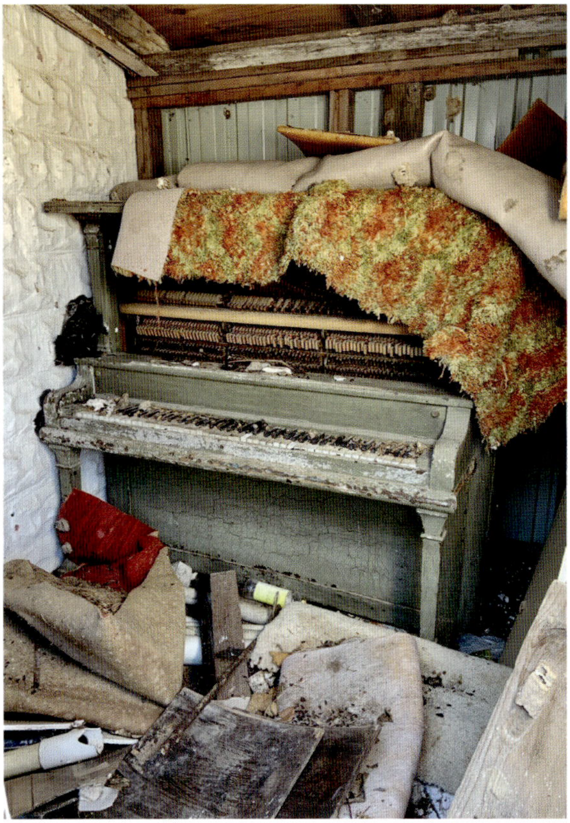

Left: Piano left inside the Full Gospel Revival Church. This would be one of two pianos that I found while going through town, March 2019.

Below: Inside the one room Full Gospel Revival Church, March 2019.

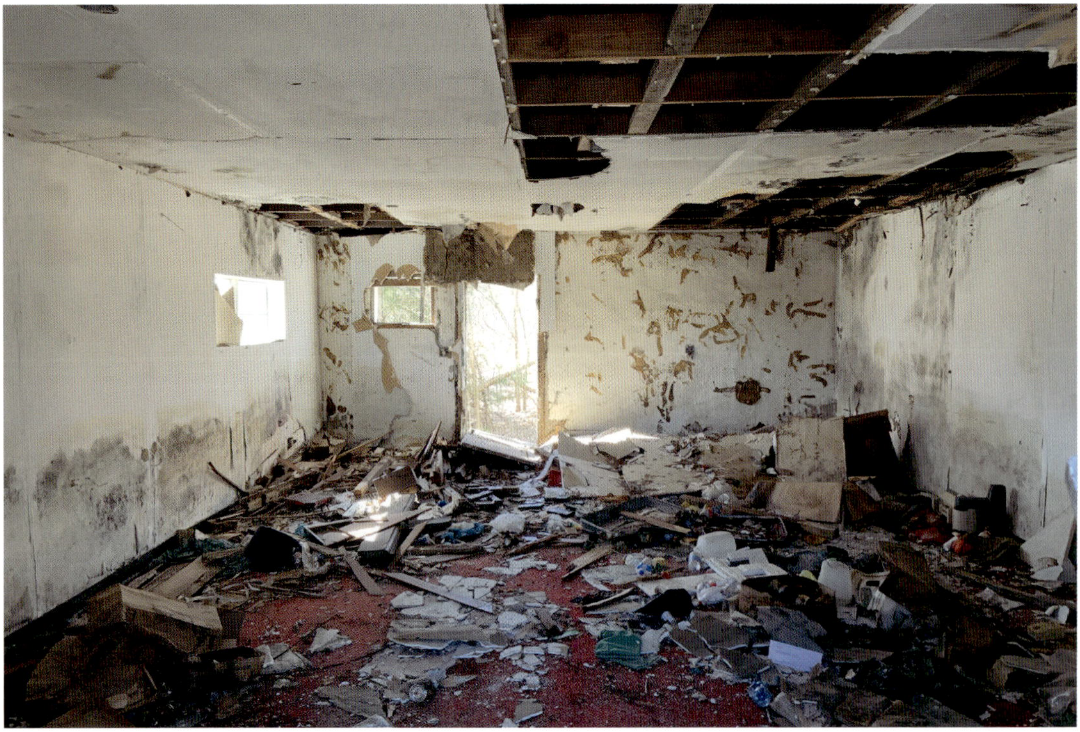

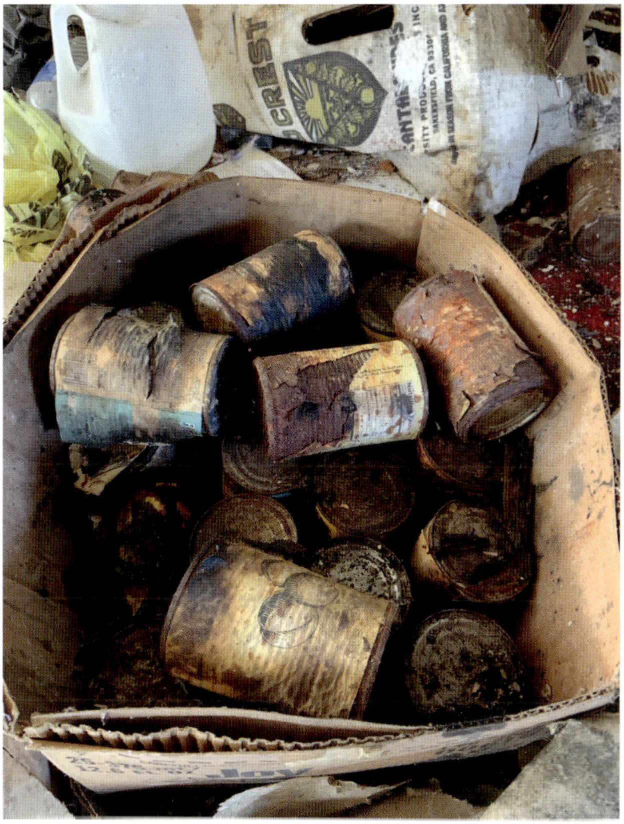

Right: One of the many boxes of rusted canned goods inside the church, March 2019.

Below: Some of the VHS tapes that was scattered all over the floor inside the Full Gospel Revival Church, March 2019.

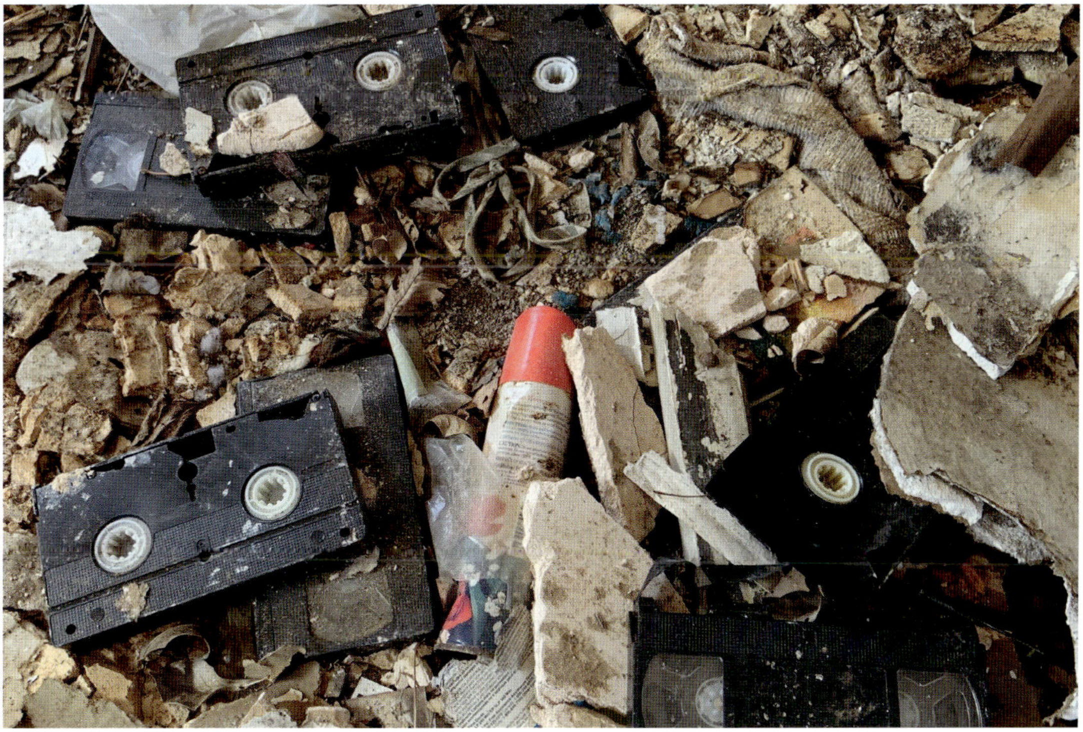

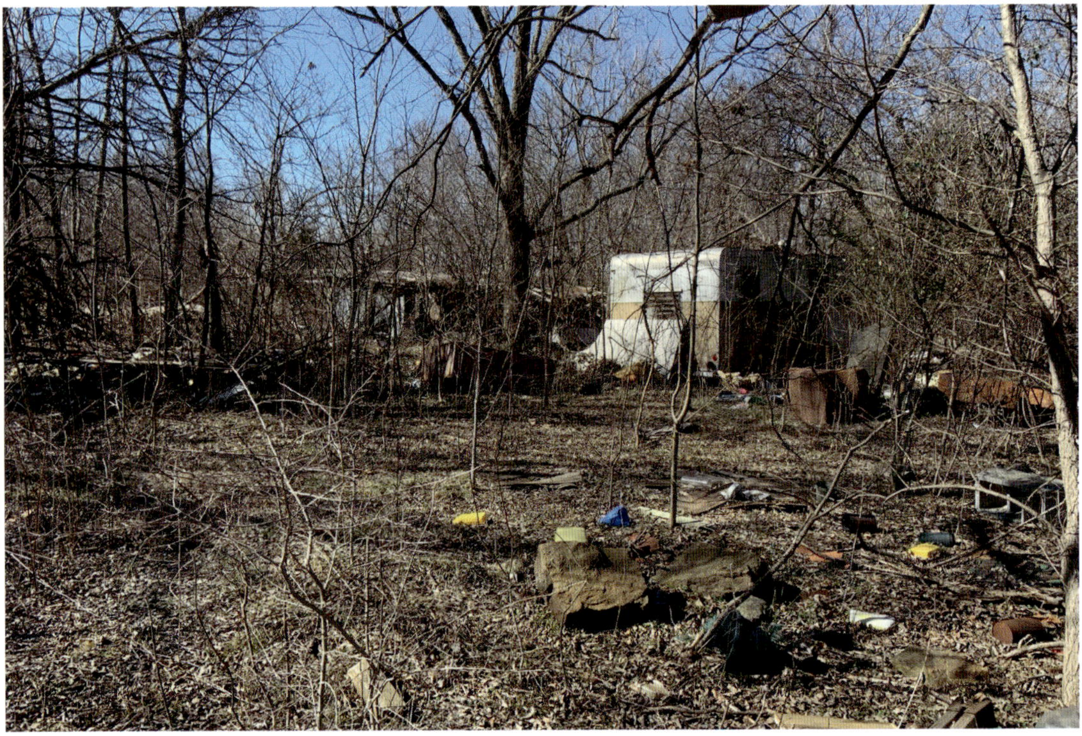

Walking out the back door of the Full Gospel Revival Church there was a small trailer and shed, March 2019.

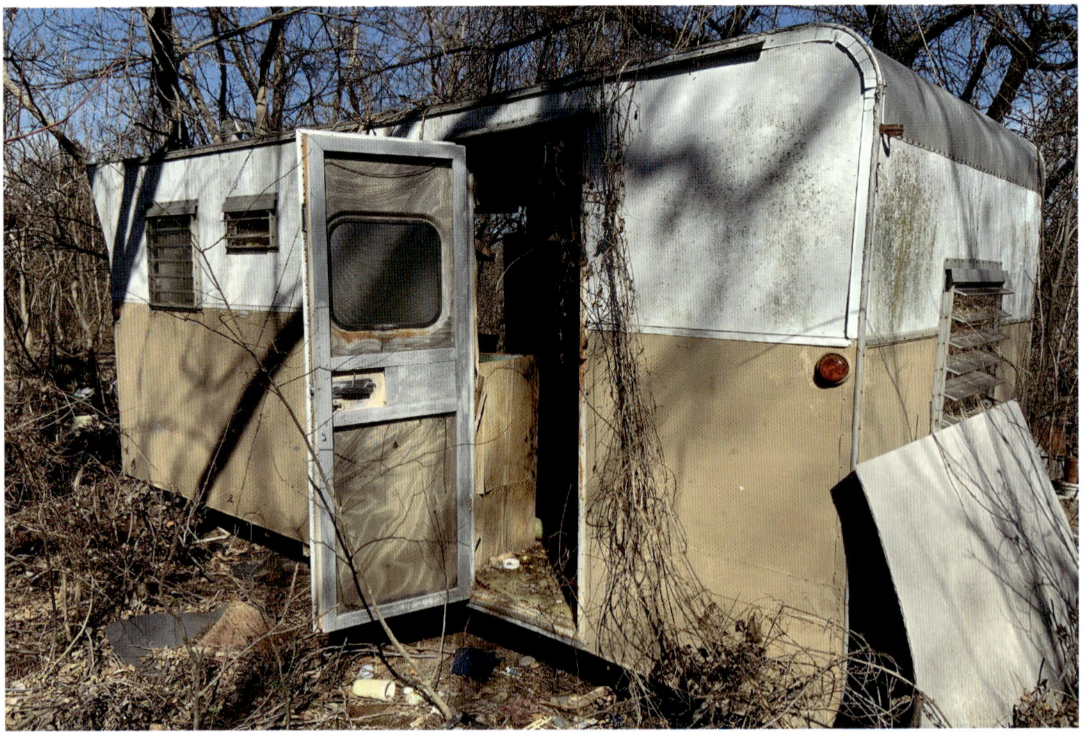

Vintage camper located behind the Full Gopel Revival Church, March 2019.

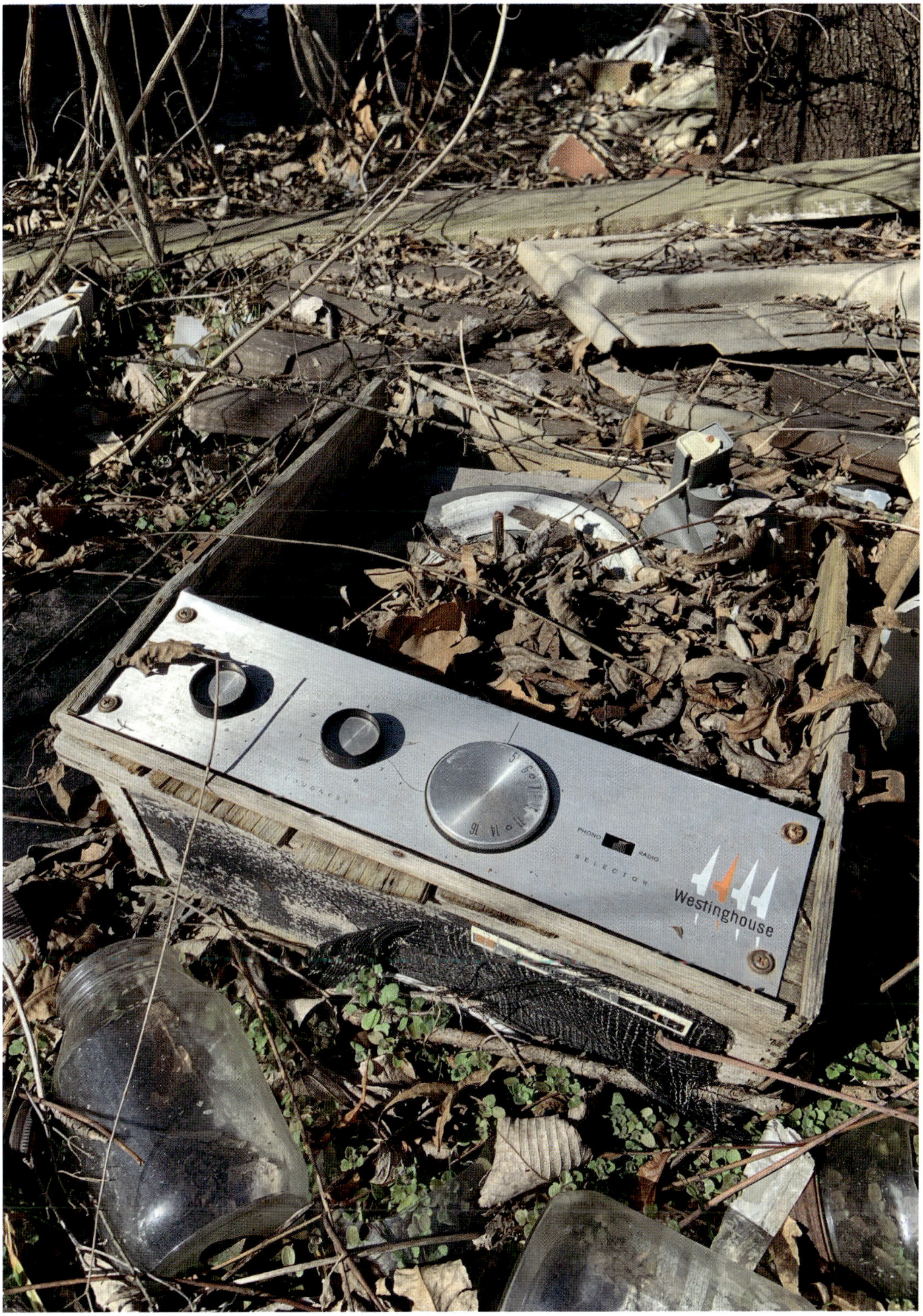

A Westinghouse record player and glass jars laying outside the vintage camper, March 2019.

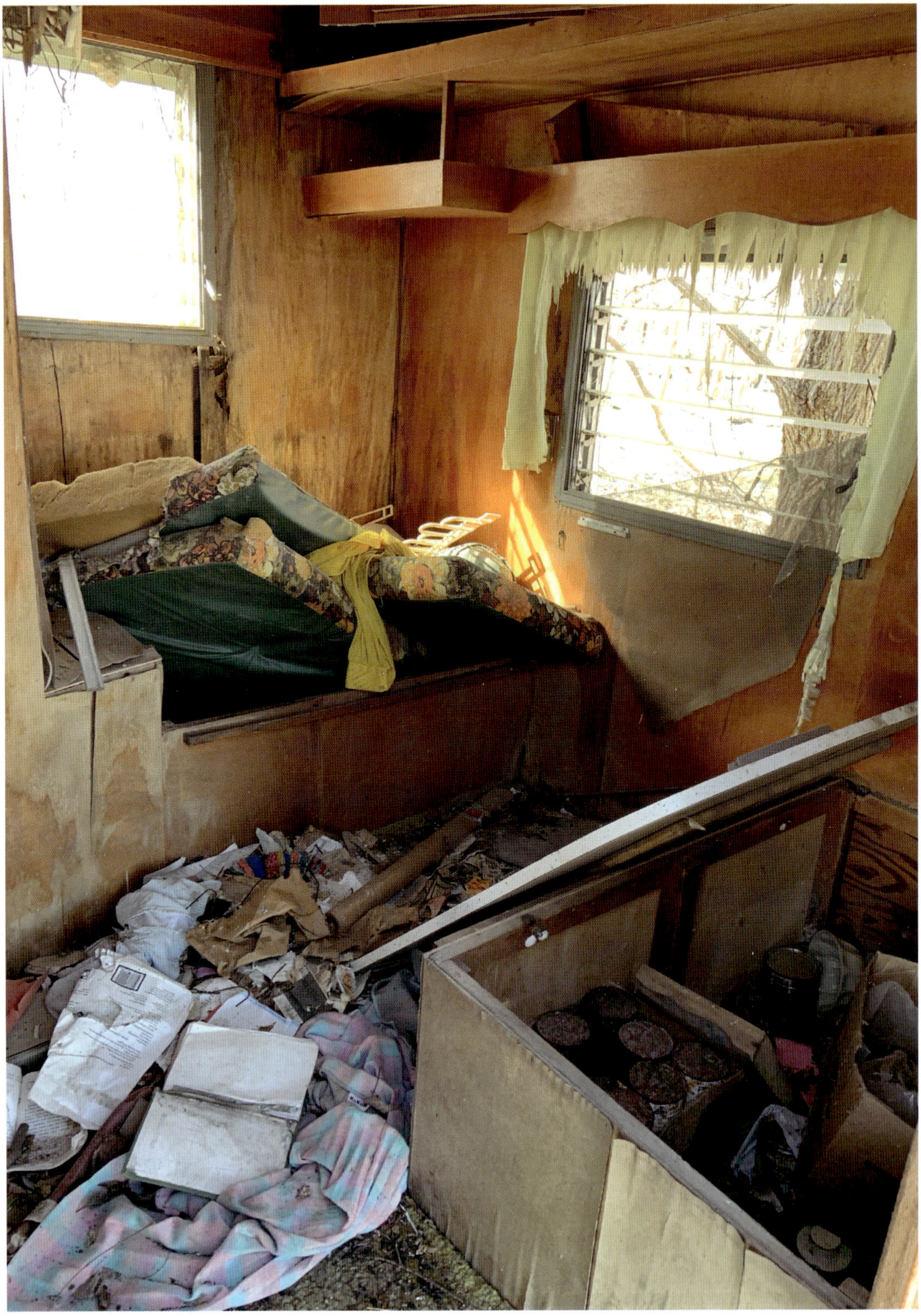

You can still see the canned goods in the compartment under the table inside the vintage camper, March 2019.

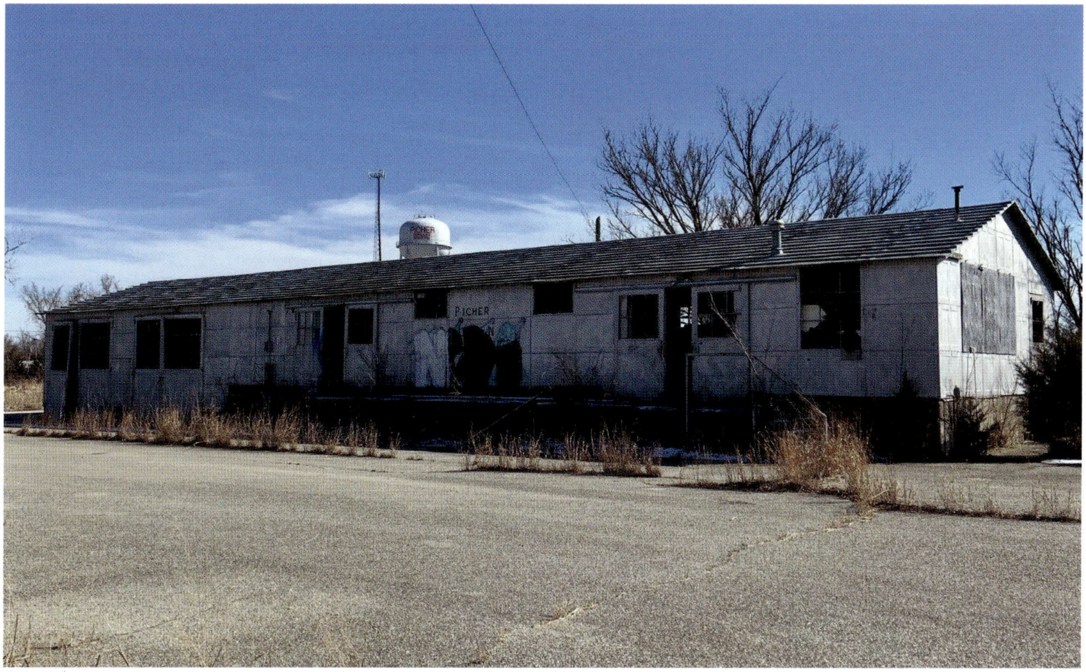

Located behind the former G&J's Gorilla Cage restaurant on the corner of Connell Avenue and "A" Street is the Picher Auction house. I was only able to find out what this building was based on 2014 Street View searches, March 2019.

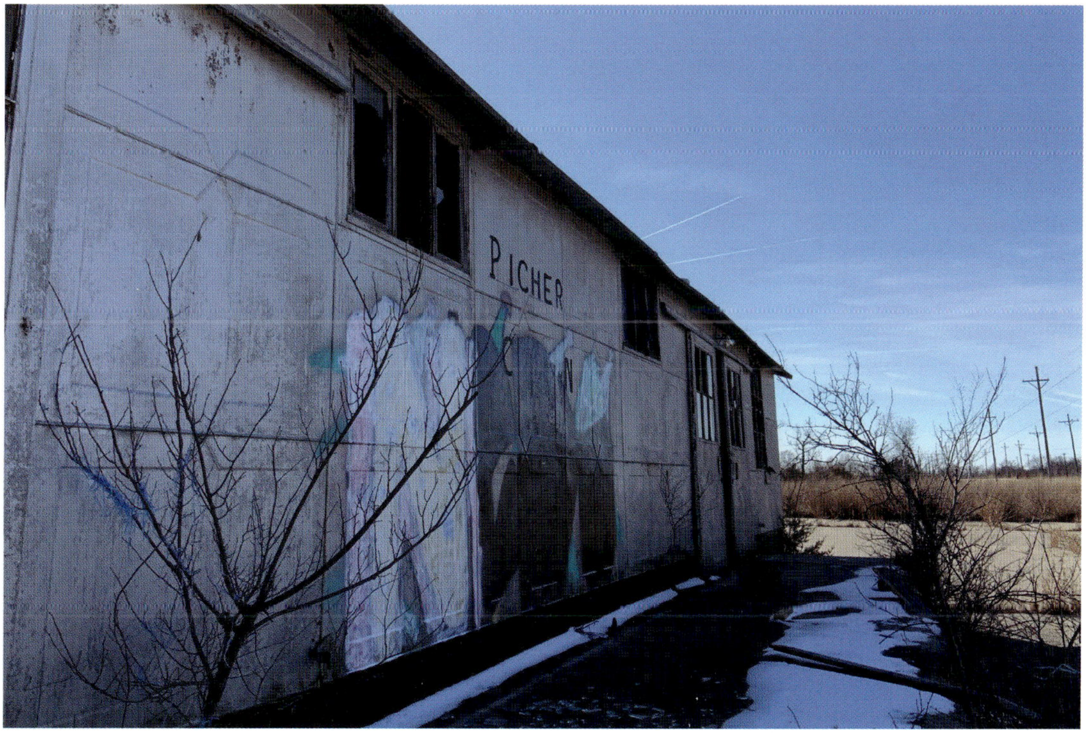

Only the word "Picher" can be read on the front of the Picher Auction house, March 2019.

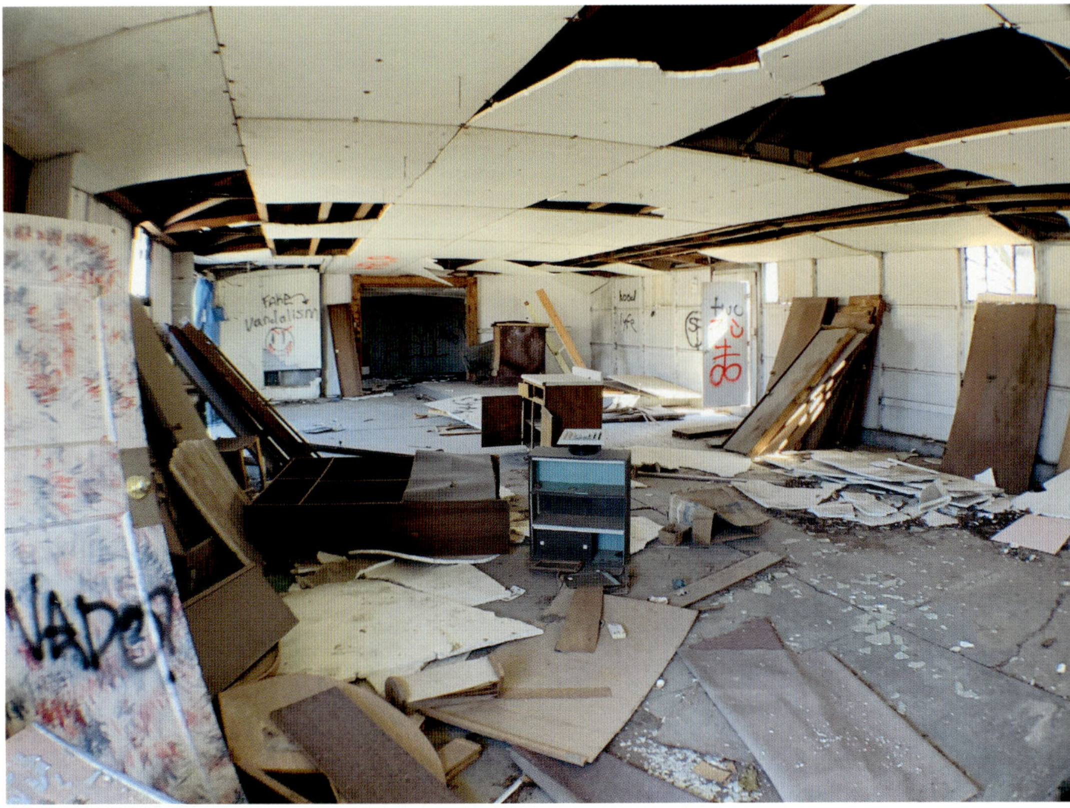

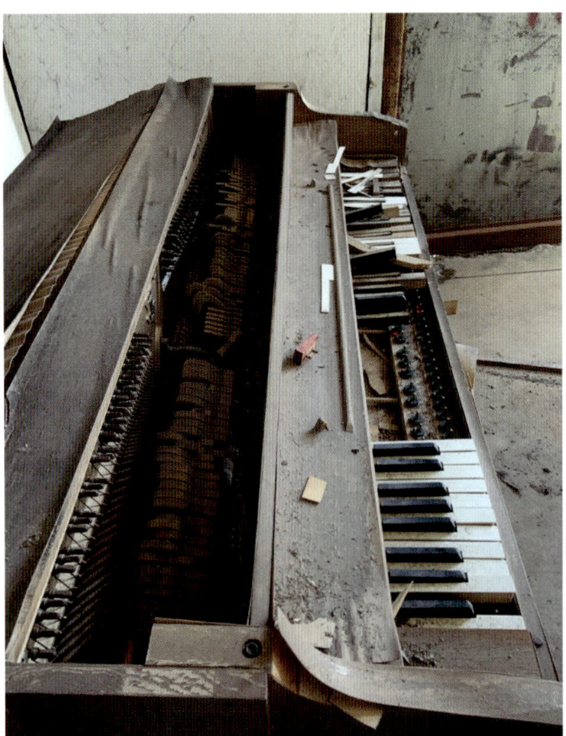

Above: Inside the Picher Auction house, March 2019.

Left: Broken piano found inside the Picher Auction house, March 2019.

through the collapsed walls. The remaining houses were safe enough to enter, but what was inside made me kind of sad. These families did not take much of anything. Holiday cards, unopened mail, family photos, and kid's toys were just left as if these people had no time to grab anything. Calendars and décor still hung on the walls. A full roll of paper towels was still in its holder in the kitchen. Toothbrushes covered in years of dust were still placed nicely in their holder. I thought, these people had plenty of time, why would they leave such personal and irreplaceable things behind? The whole trip was a sad realization because of the level of damage that has been done to the land, environment, and hundreds of residents, including children, over the decades. The left-behind personal belongings were just the tip of the iceberg. There I was walking through what I felt was a twisted memorial to big business using up everything Picher and its people had to offer and leaving behind long-term damage. Even though the damage is long term, it does not mean that it cannot be corrected.

I wondered if the owners of everything left behind missed any of these personal things. How many kids were missing their favorite bear or baby doll? Seeing all of this was a rush of emotions, it made me think about if I had to pack up and leave. Sad because I would have to leave possibly the only thing I have ever known, but on the other hand, happy for a second chance at a new life in a new place.

As for the clean-up efforts, I saw a lot of signs throughout town that the area was part of a government clean up. In addition to the signs, there was also numerous trucks leaving the piles with full loads of chat, off to be refined. In the more residential areas, there was some heavy equipment and men working to clean up downed trees, trash, and debris. However, these are only baby steps to clean up the decades of damage and contamination that has driven away people and made the local waters run a rusty color. It is the ultimate goal of the Quapaw Nation and all government agencies involved to have all the chat and contamination cleaned up, abandoned mines filled in to avoid future sinkholes, and clean water that is safe for use and consumption; however, they are finding out that more money is needed and the magnitude of this large-scale project is overwhelming. Overwhelmed but not discouraged, positive results are coming in. The year 2008 proved to be a big one for the cleaning of local waters. A ten-pond filtration system started purifying the water from the mines and lead and zinc run off. These ponds clean the water before it is filtered back into Tar Creek. In addition to the filtration system, contaminated dirt from the surrounding homes are being tested for lead and zinc, then removed and replaced with contaminate free dirt in an effort to minimize the spreading of contaminates. With the implementing of these clean-up efforts, also comes the ongoing monitoring and retesting of the waters and soils, to ensure the progress keeps going in the right direction.

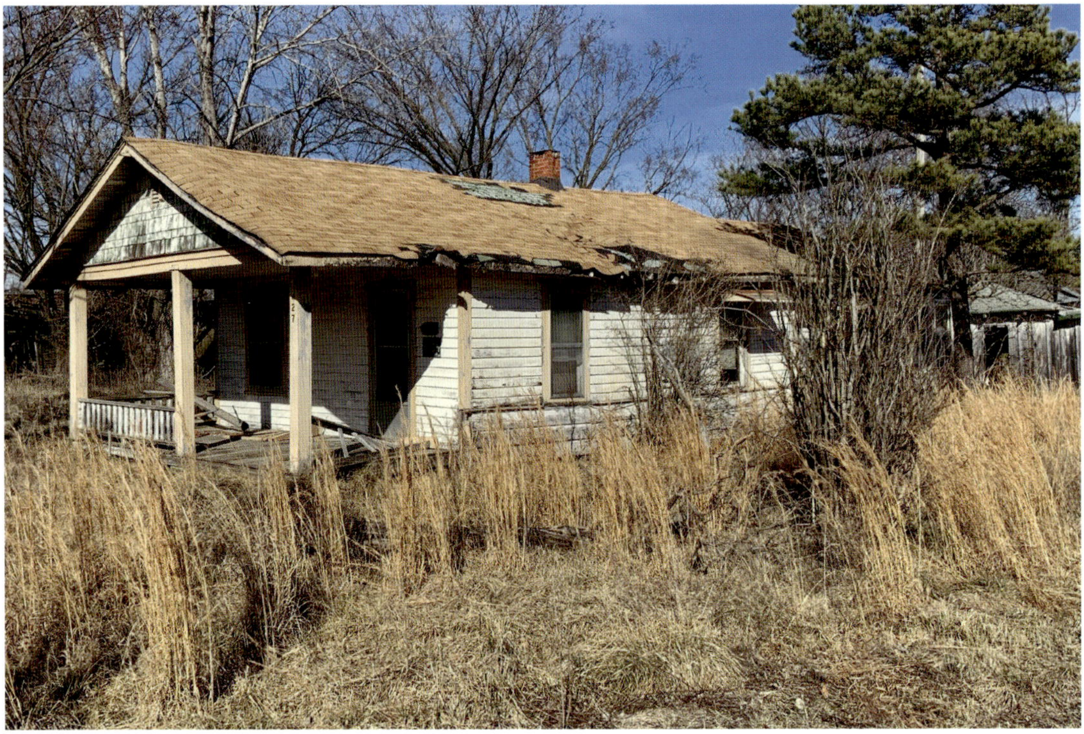

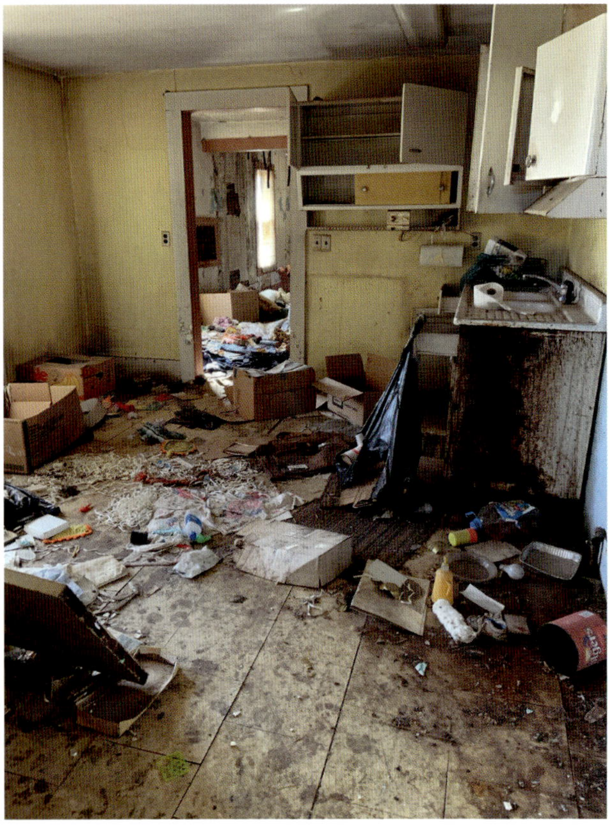

Above: Based on the mail that was left all over the floor of this house, Claude Best lived here, March 2019.

Left: Kitchen inside Claude's house, March 2019.

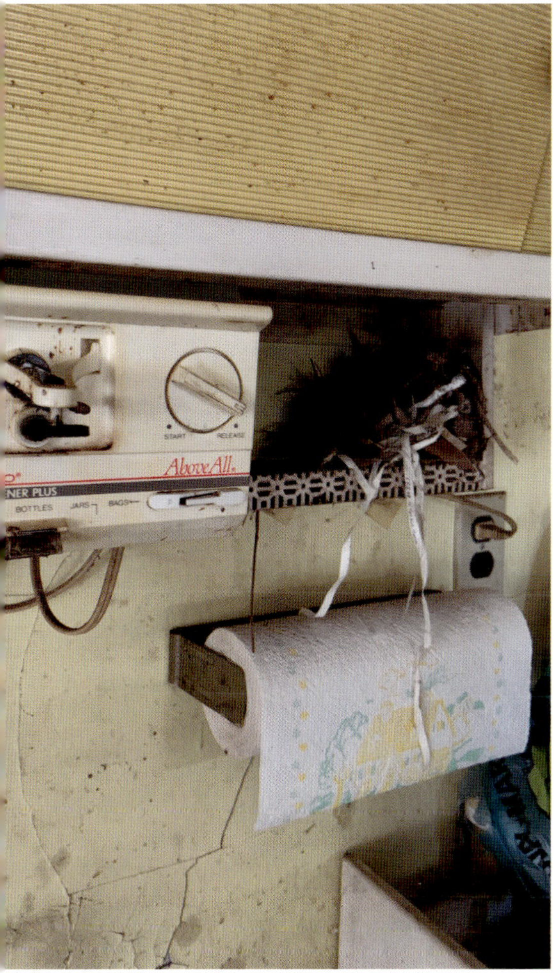

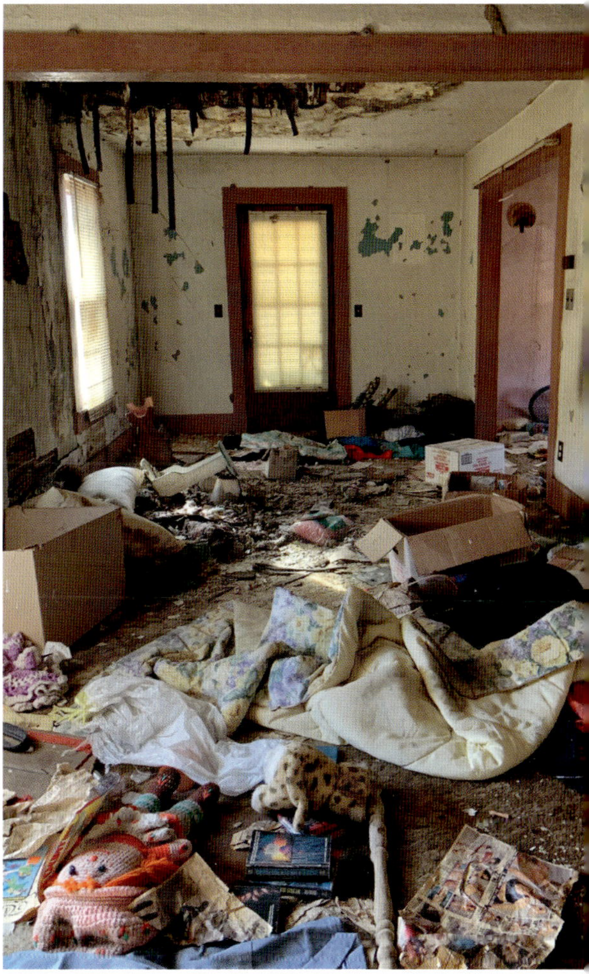

Above left: Next to the can opener, a bird has built a nest in the shelf above the roll of paper towels that still hang in the kitchen, March 2019.

Above right: Living room inside Claude's house. Personal belongings left behind, only to be thrown all over the house, March 2019.

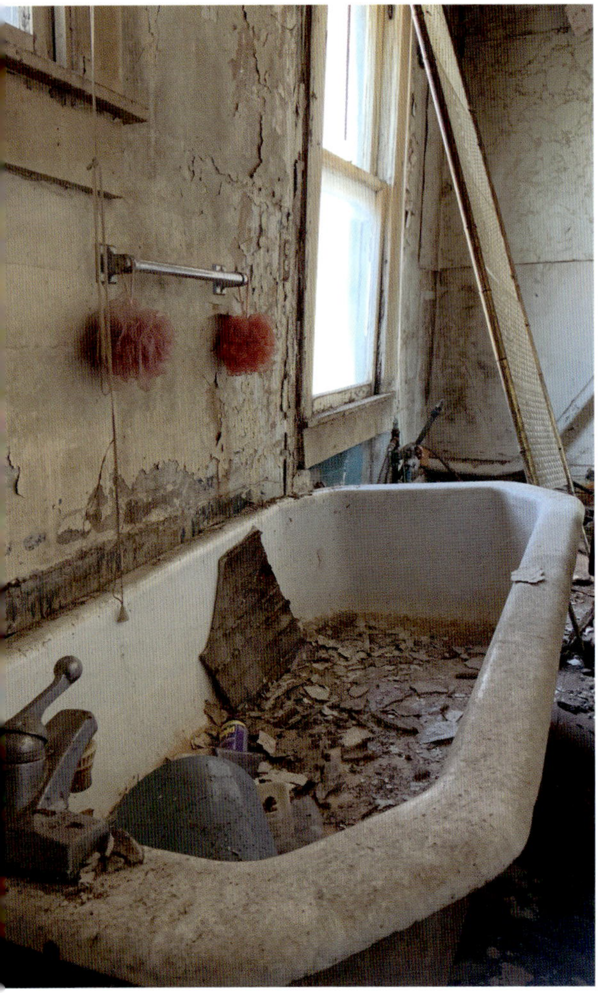

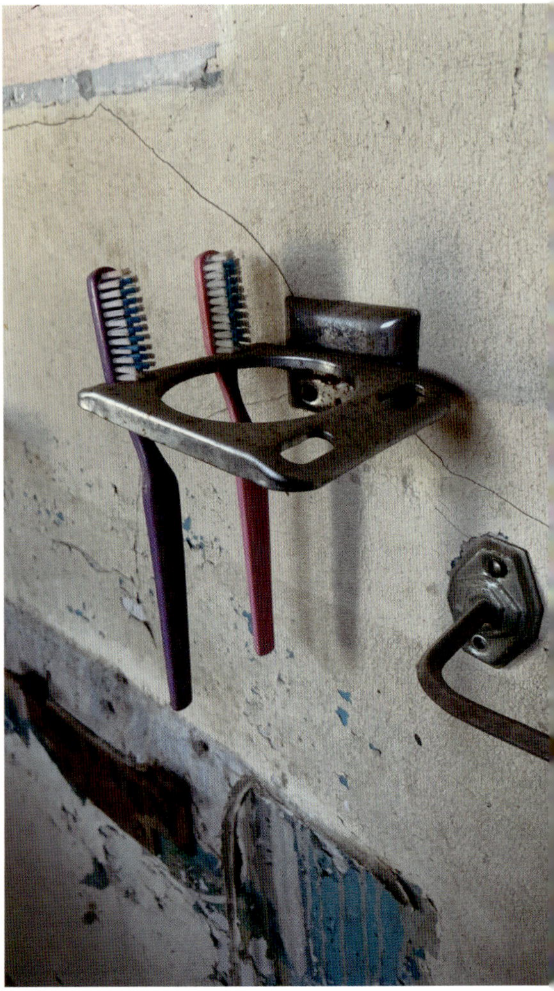

Above left: Loofahs still hang on the towel rack in the bathroom of Claude's house, March 2019.

Above right: Toothbrushes still in the toothbrush holder in the bathroom of Claude's house, March 2019.

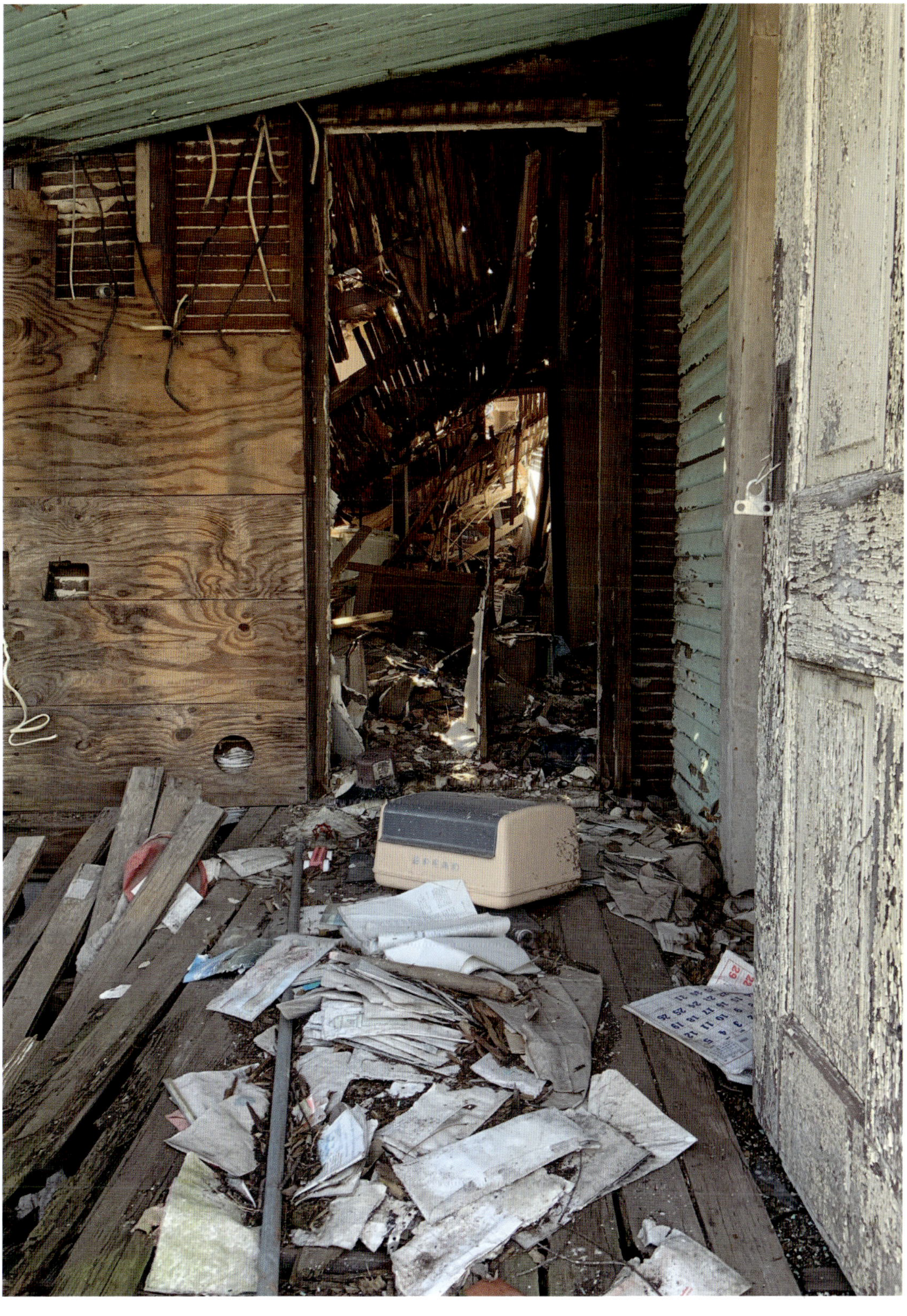

Standing at the back door of a collapsing house, March 2019.

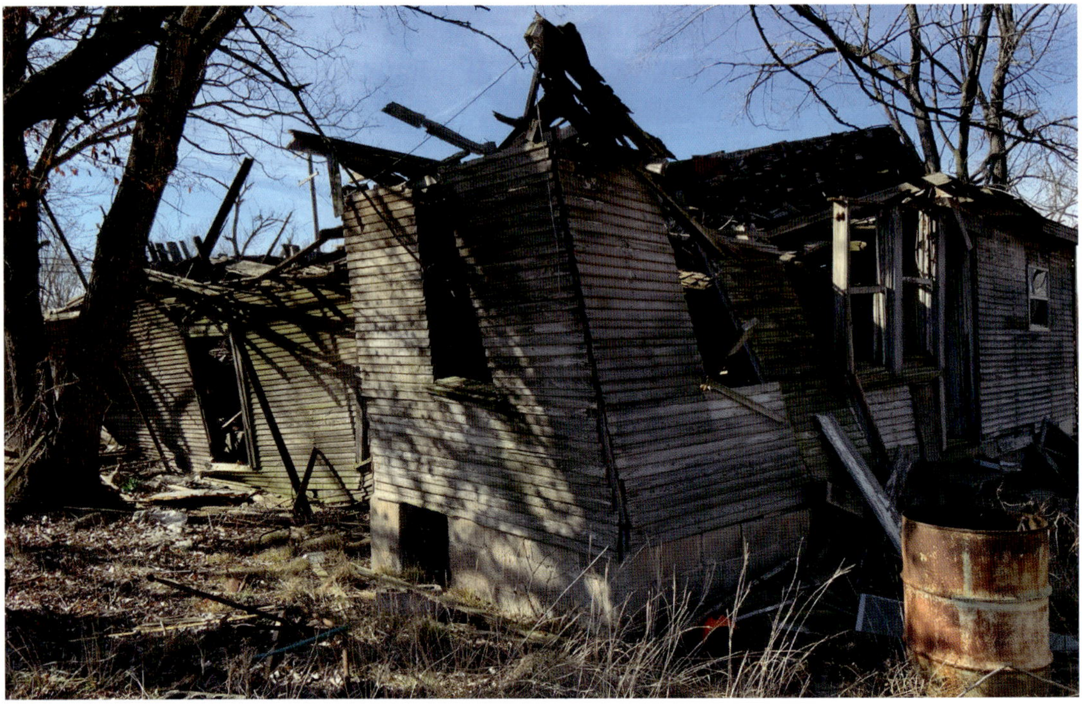

Another collapsing house located in Picher, March 2019.

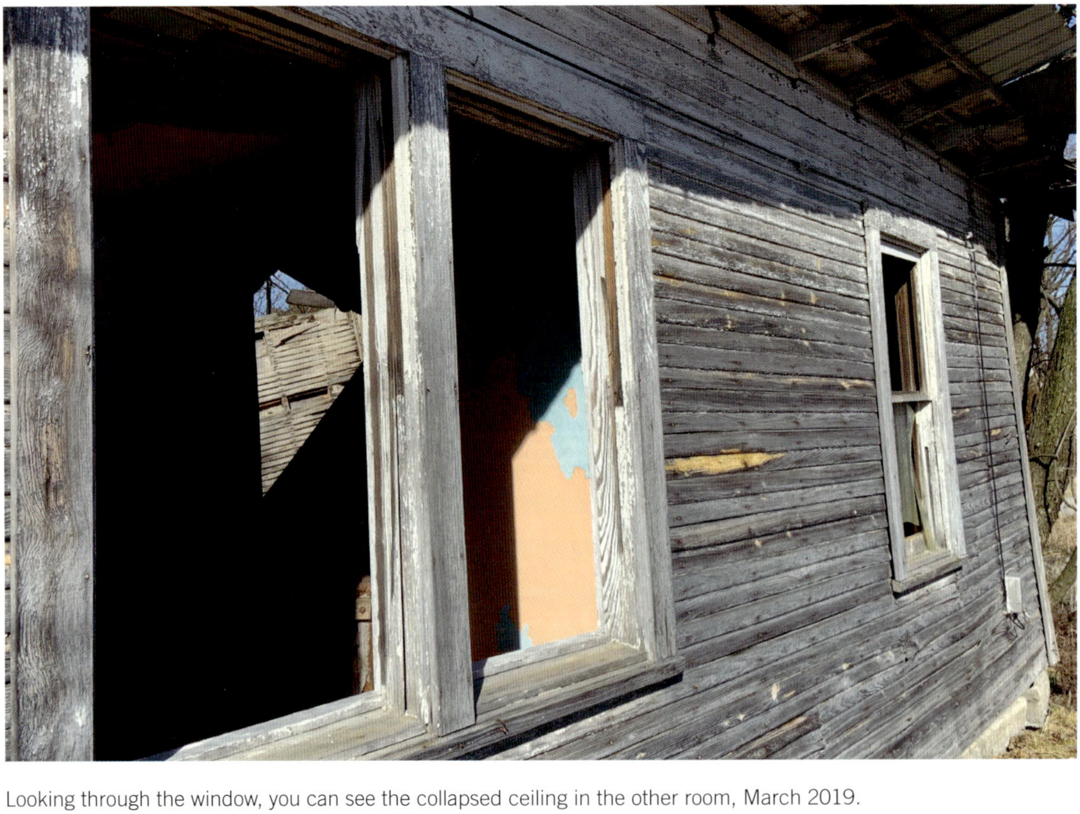

Looking through the window, you can see the collapsed ceiling in the other room, March 2019.

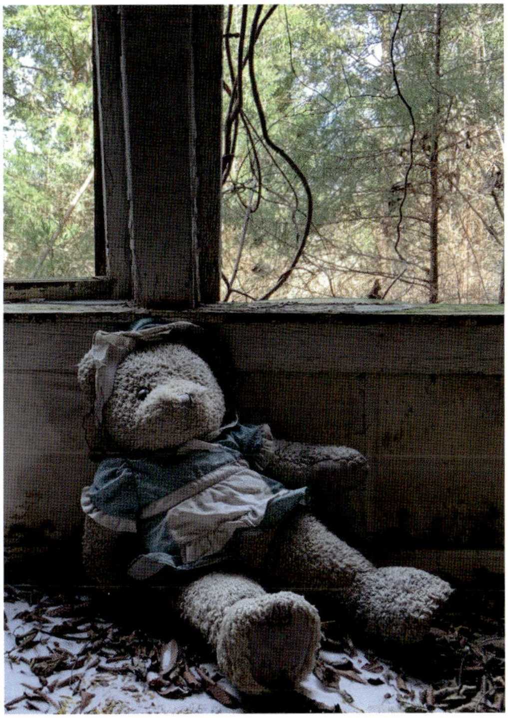

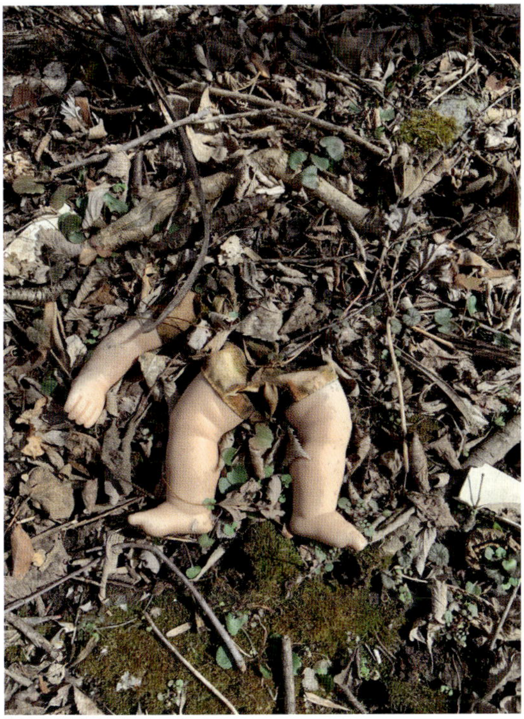

Above left: Teddy was waiting for me to return, March 2019.

Above right: Baby doll remains behind the mobile home, March 2019.

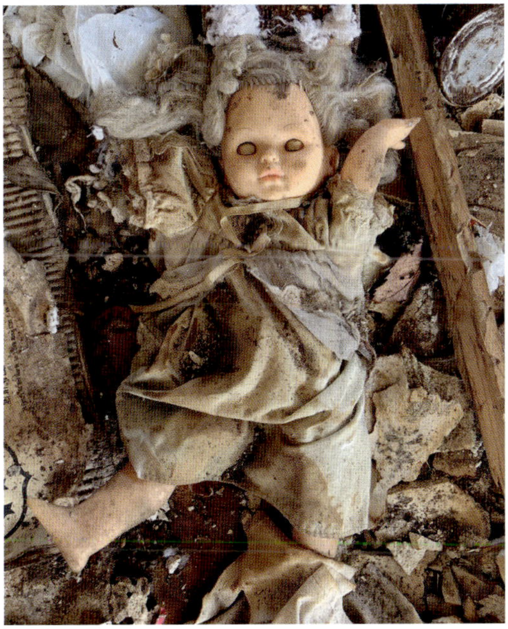

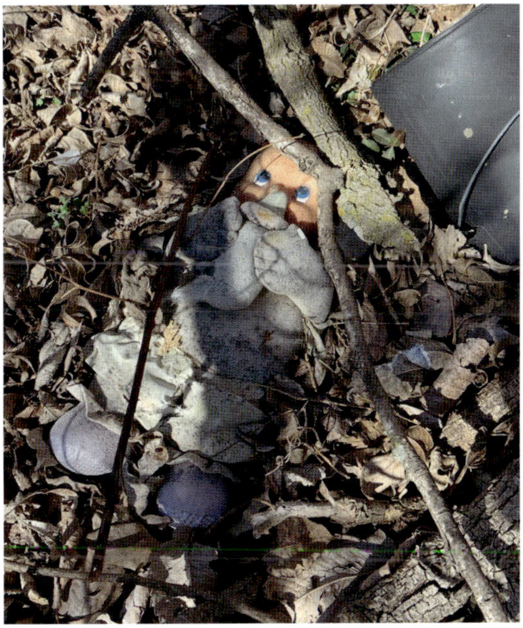

Above left: Another abandoned baby doll, March 2019.

Above right: Another lost baby doll, March 2019.

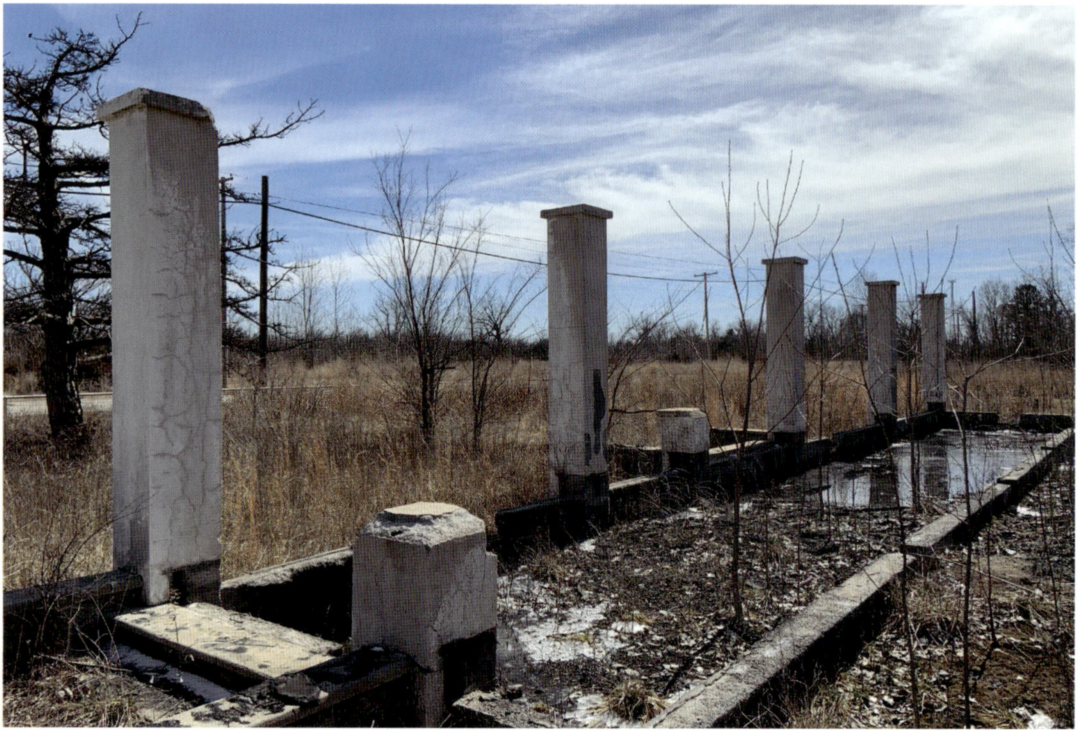

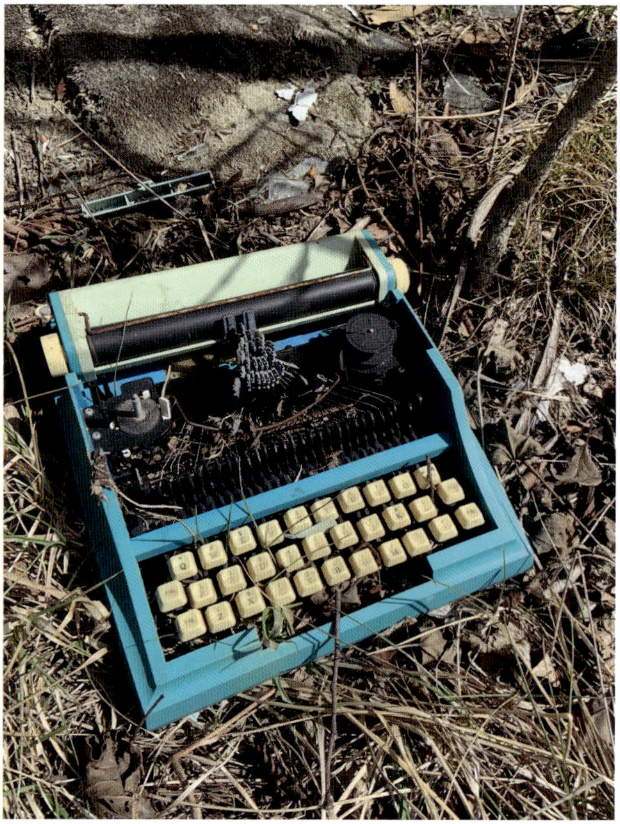

Above: Side view of the mining museum's front porch pillars, March 2019.

Left: Children's typewriter left on the ground outside a house, March 2019.

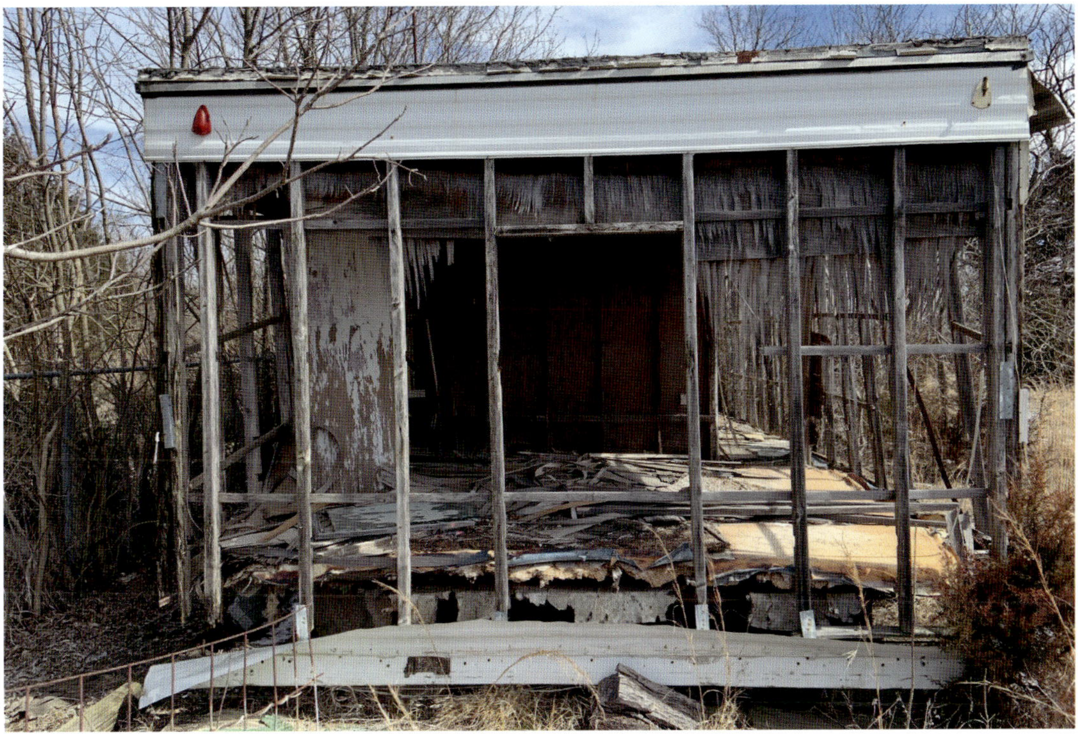

Above: End view of the mobile home with no siding, March 2019.

Right: Baby rocking bed covered with insulation from the collapsing ceiling in the living room of Claude's house, March 2019.

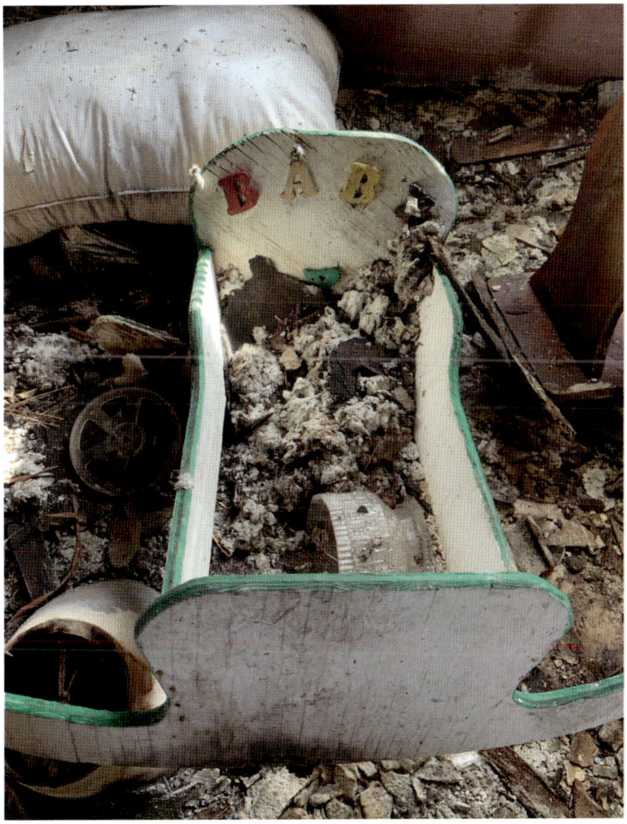

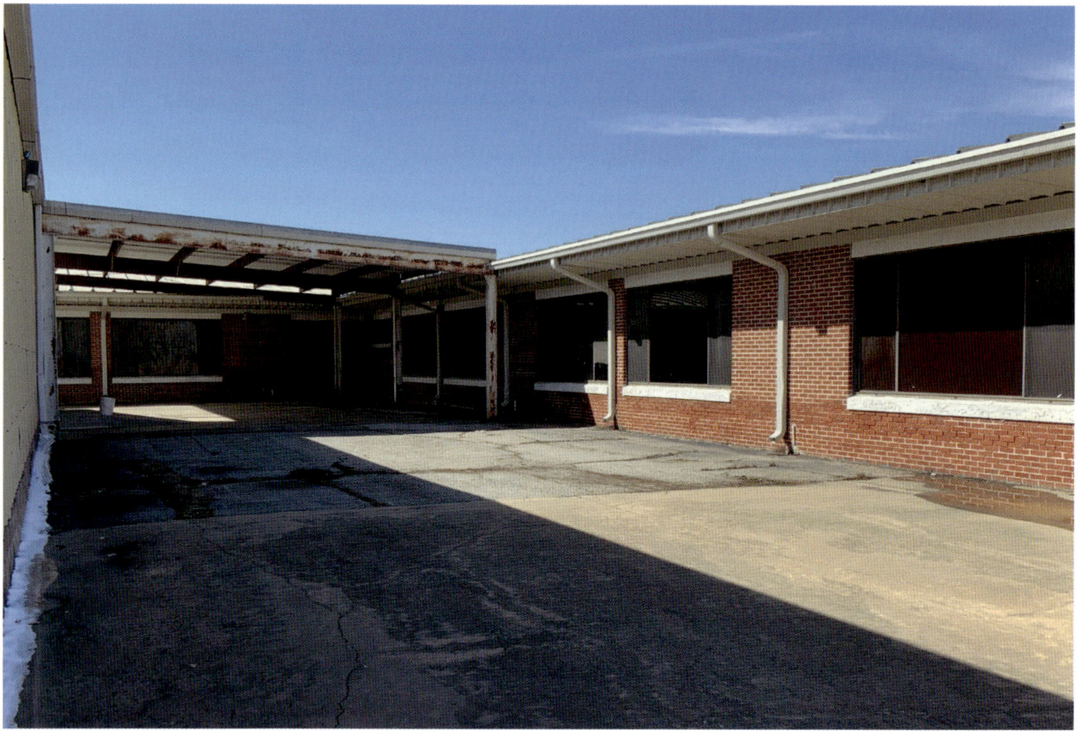

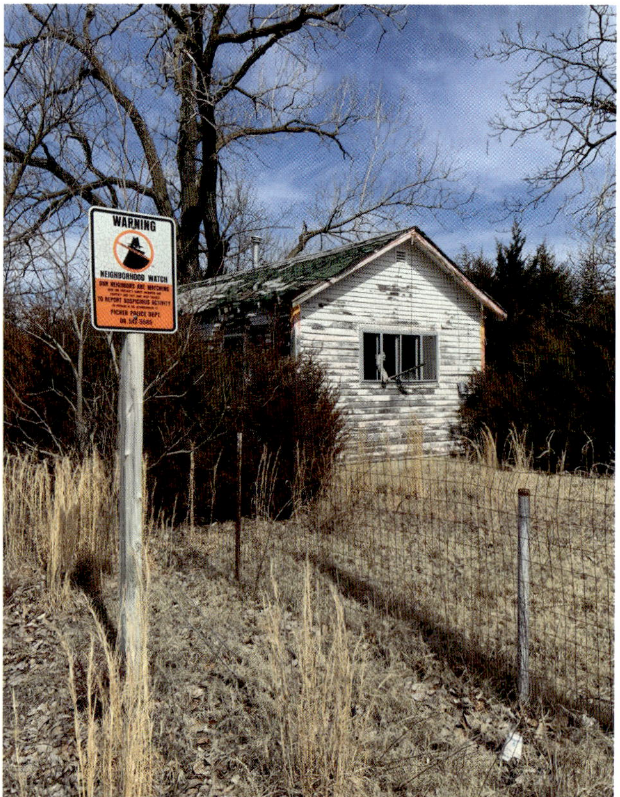
WARNING
NEIGHBORHOOD WATCH
OUR NEIGHBORS ARE WATCHING
TO REPORT SUSPICIOUS ACTIVITY
PICHER POLICE DEPT.

Above: One of the views from the back of the school, March 2019.

Left: Neighborhood watch sign still posted outside of this abandoned house, March 2019.

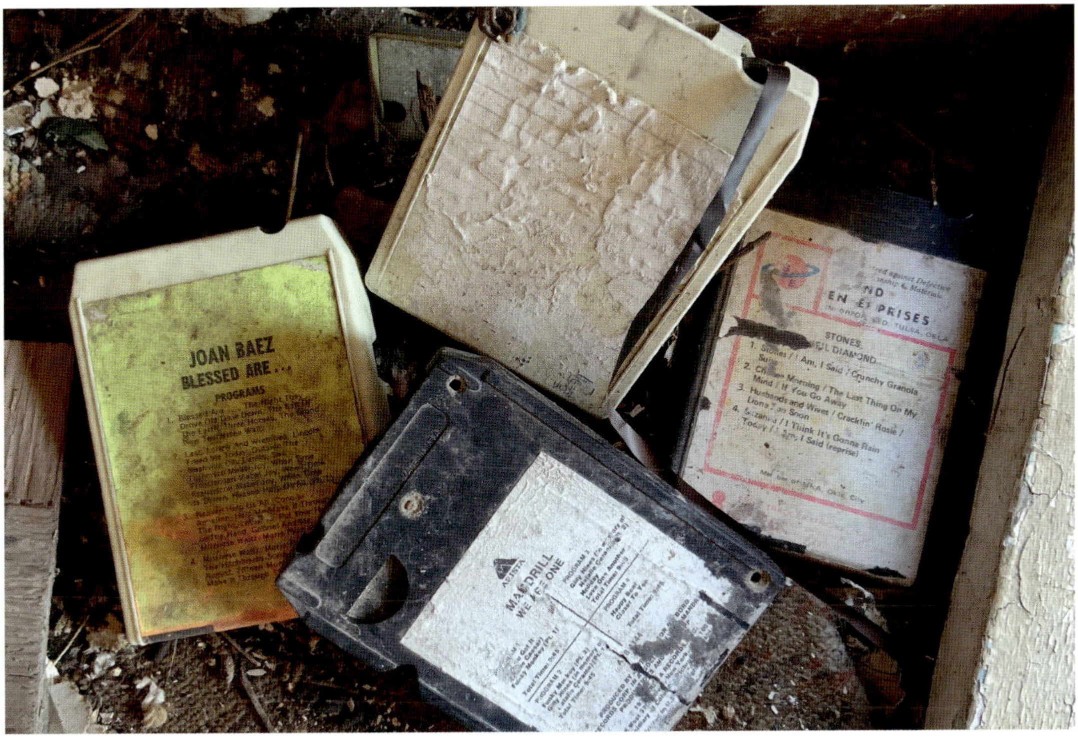

8-Tracks found on the floor in Claude's house, March 2019.

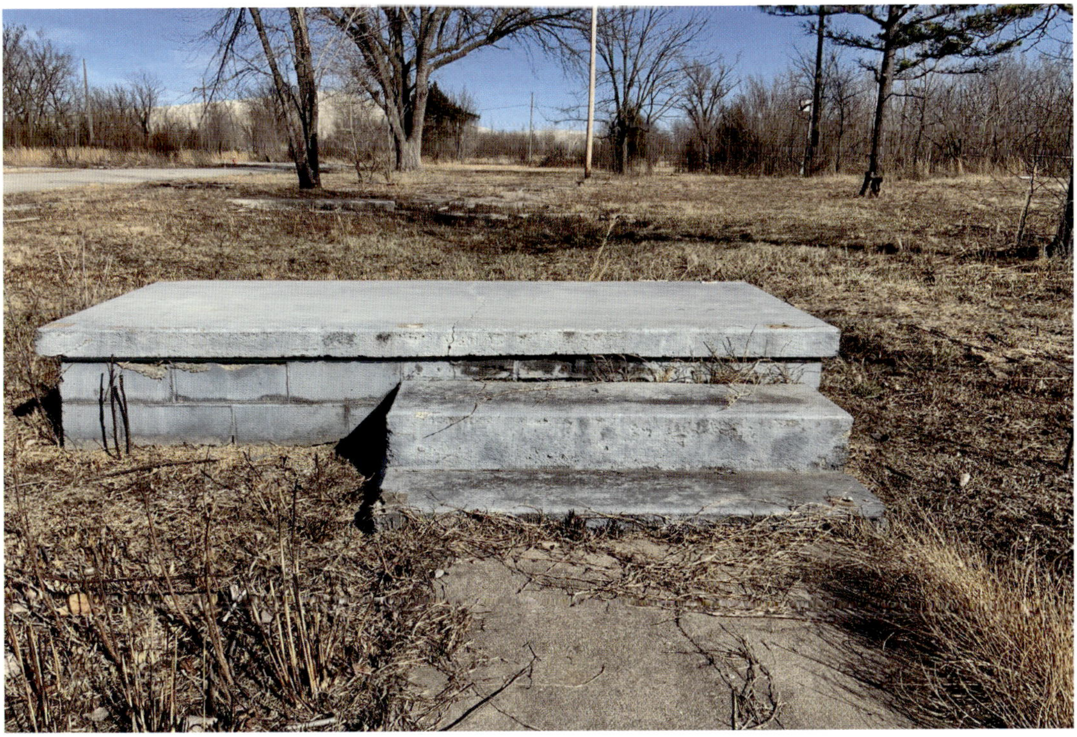

Front porch with no house, March 2019.

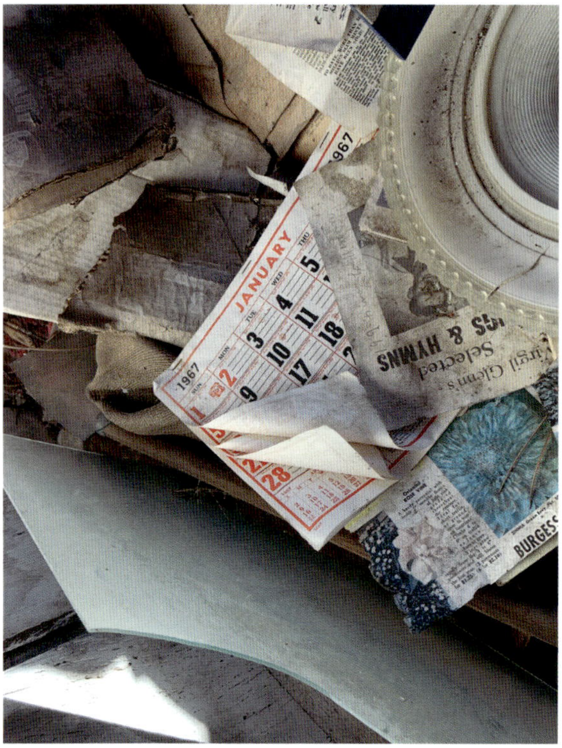

Left: Found a calendar from 1967. The same year Picher stopped all of its mining, March 2019.

Below: Shed-type shack located next to the vintage camper, March 2019.

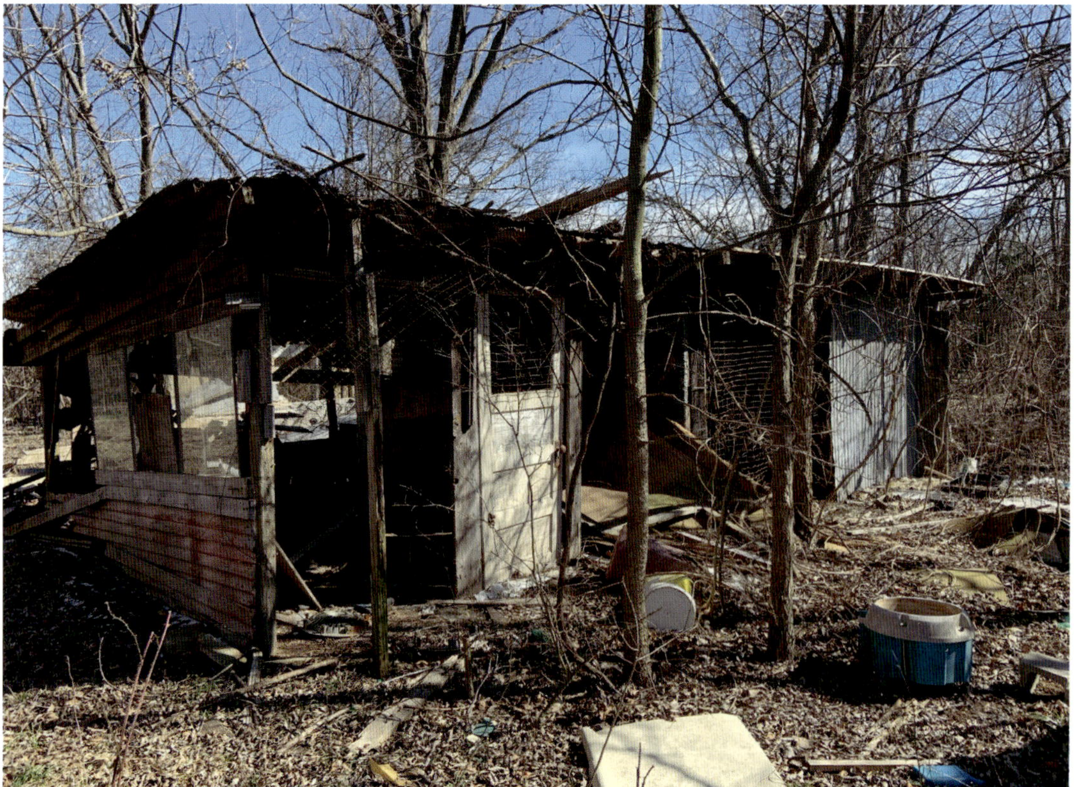

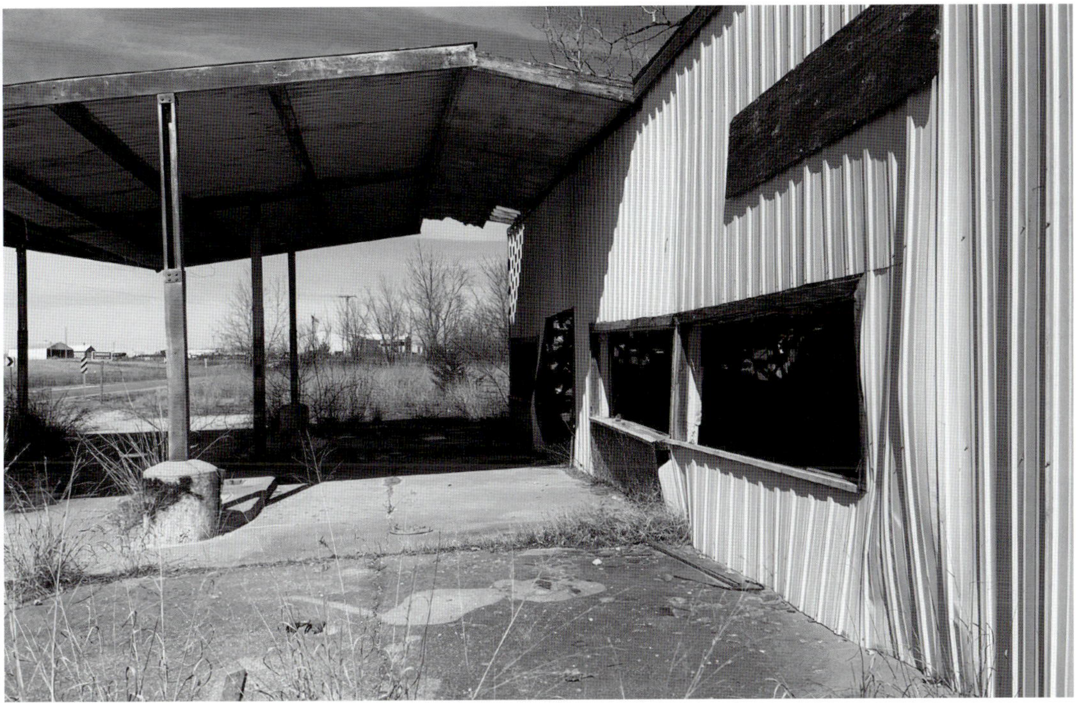

View of the gas station diner from the Oklahoma side looking into Kansas, March 2019.

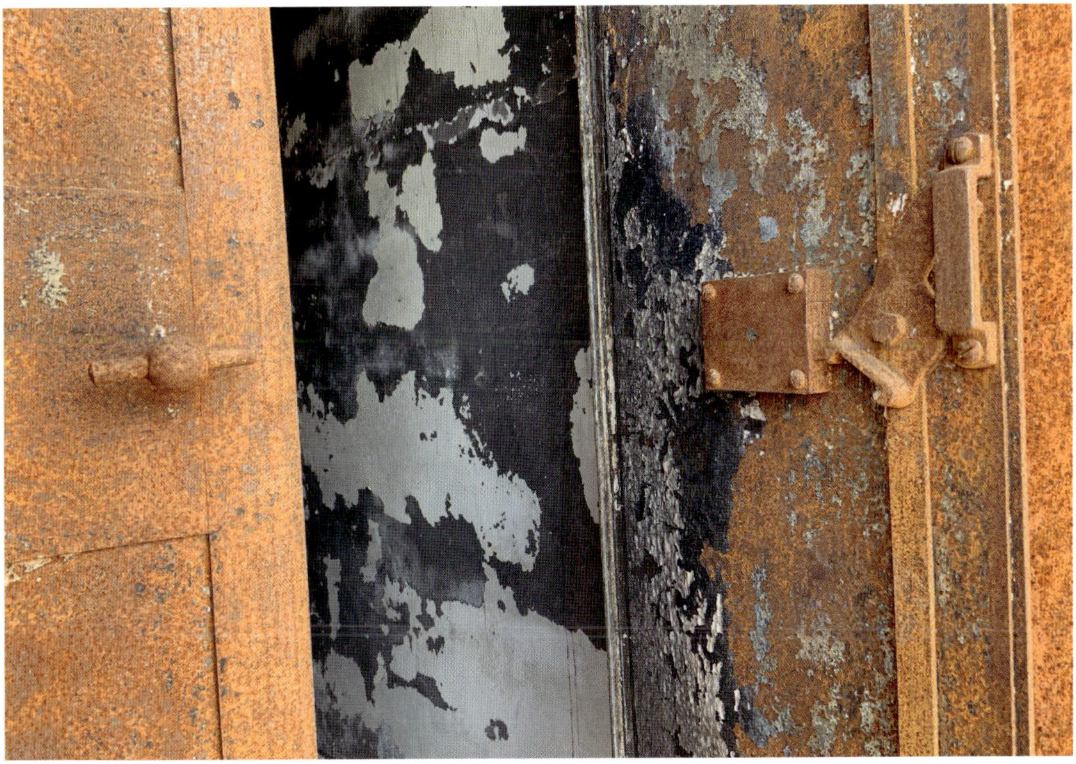

The rusted door and lock of the walk-in fireproof safe in the Picher Mining Museum, March 2019.

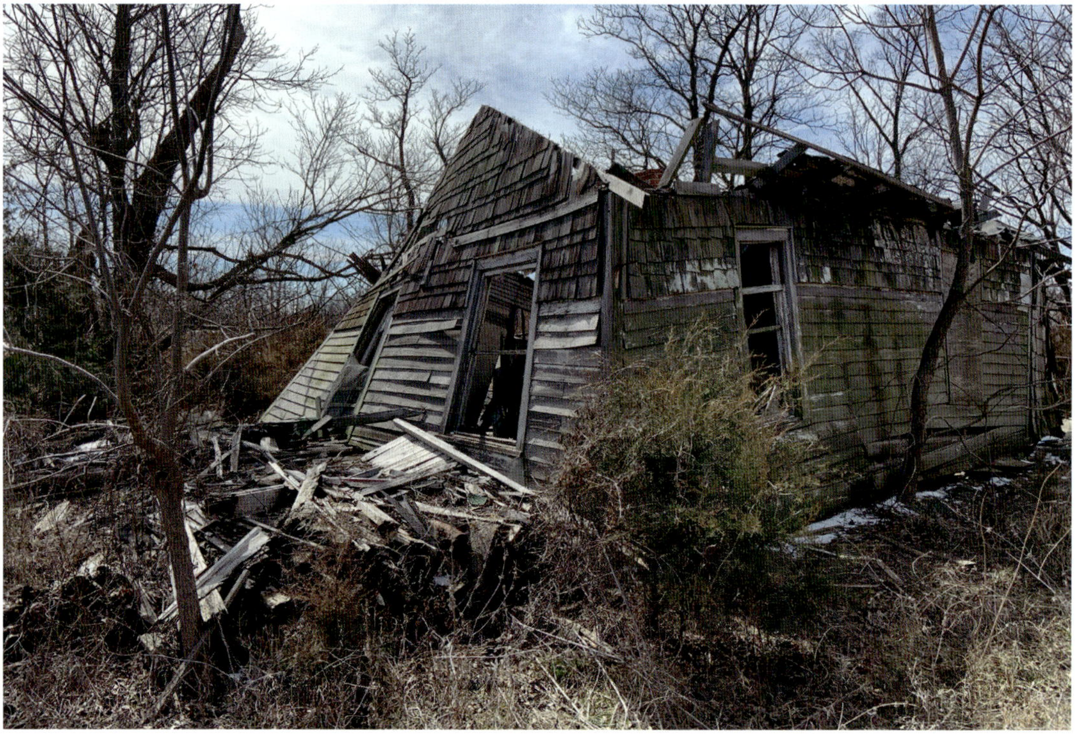

One of the many collapsing houses around Picher, March 2019.

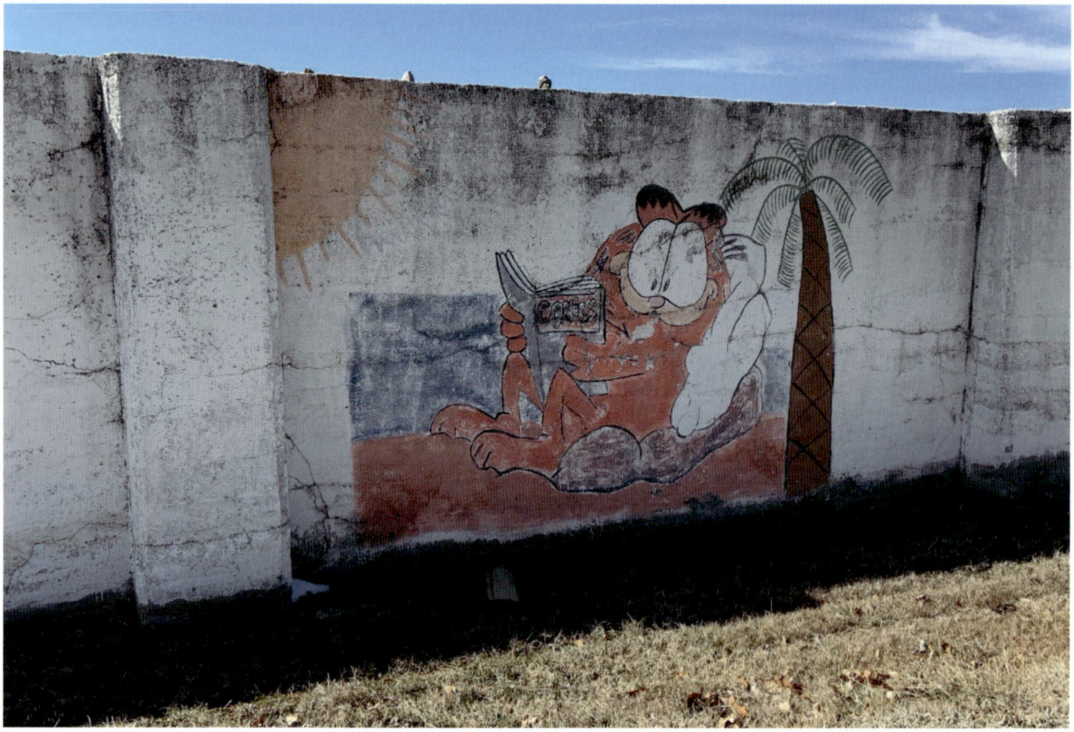

On the back of the track wall, was this completely random painting of Garfield relaxing on the beach, March 2019.

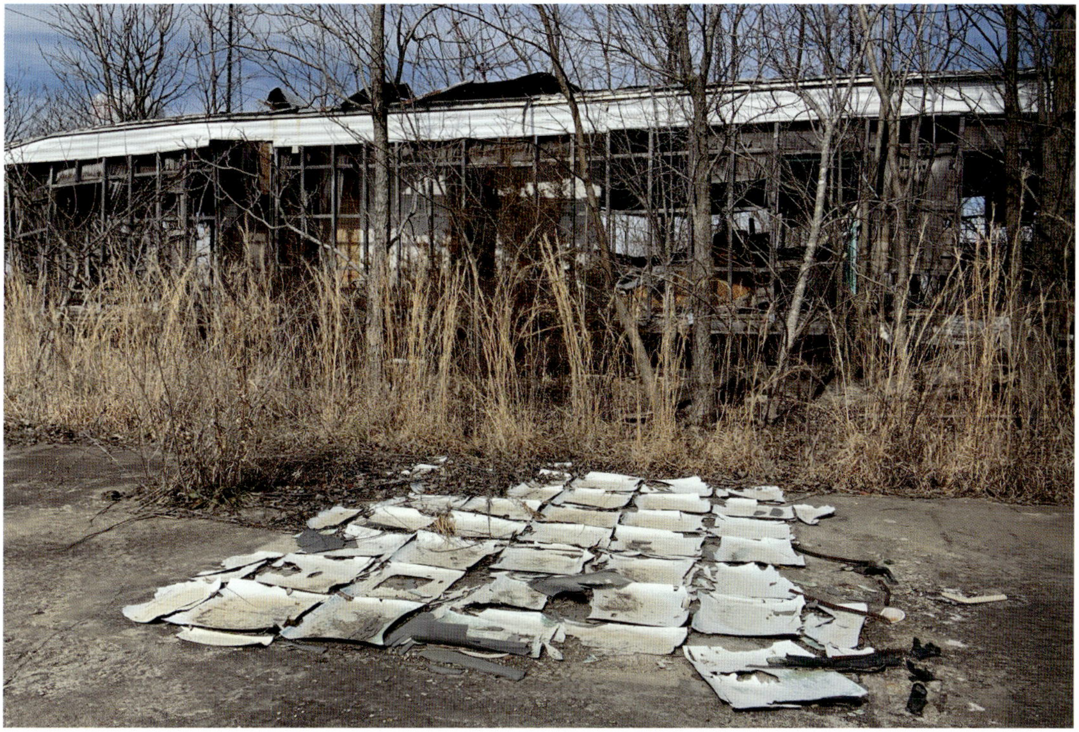

Next to the frame of a mobile home is the foundation and floor tiles of the neighboring house, March 2019.

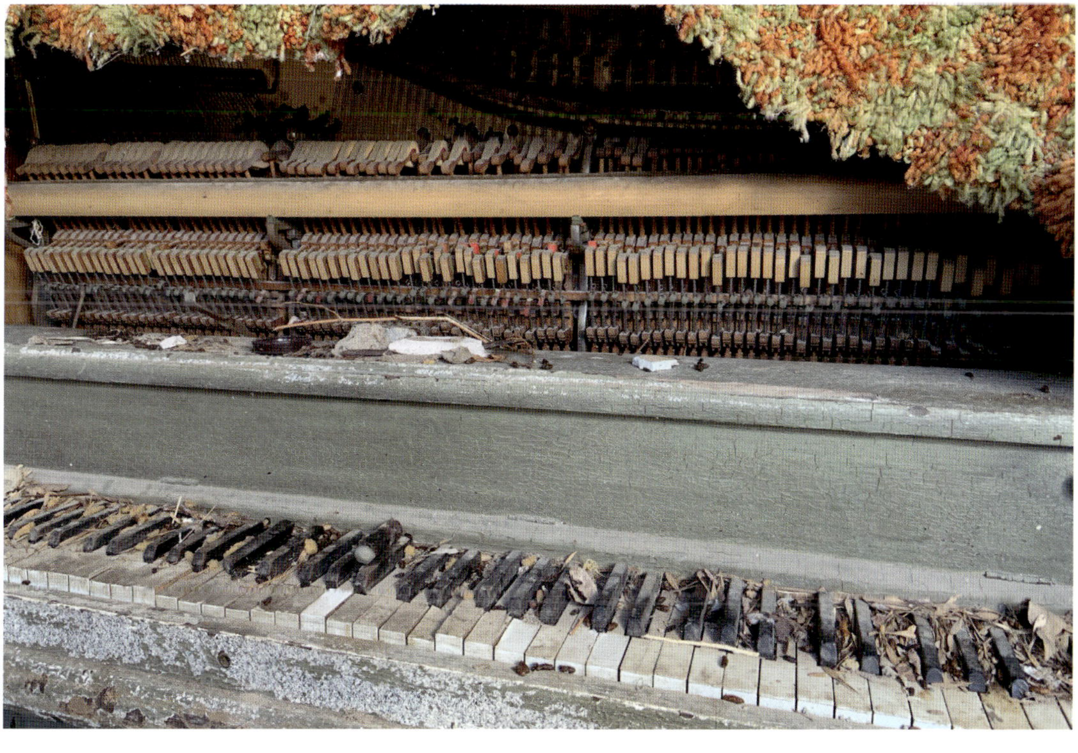

Close up of the piano left behind in the Full Gospel Revival Church. Some of the key still played, March 2019.

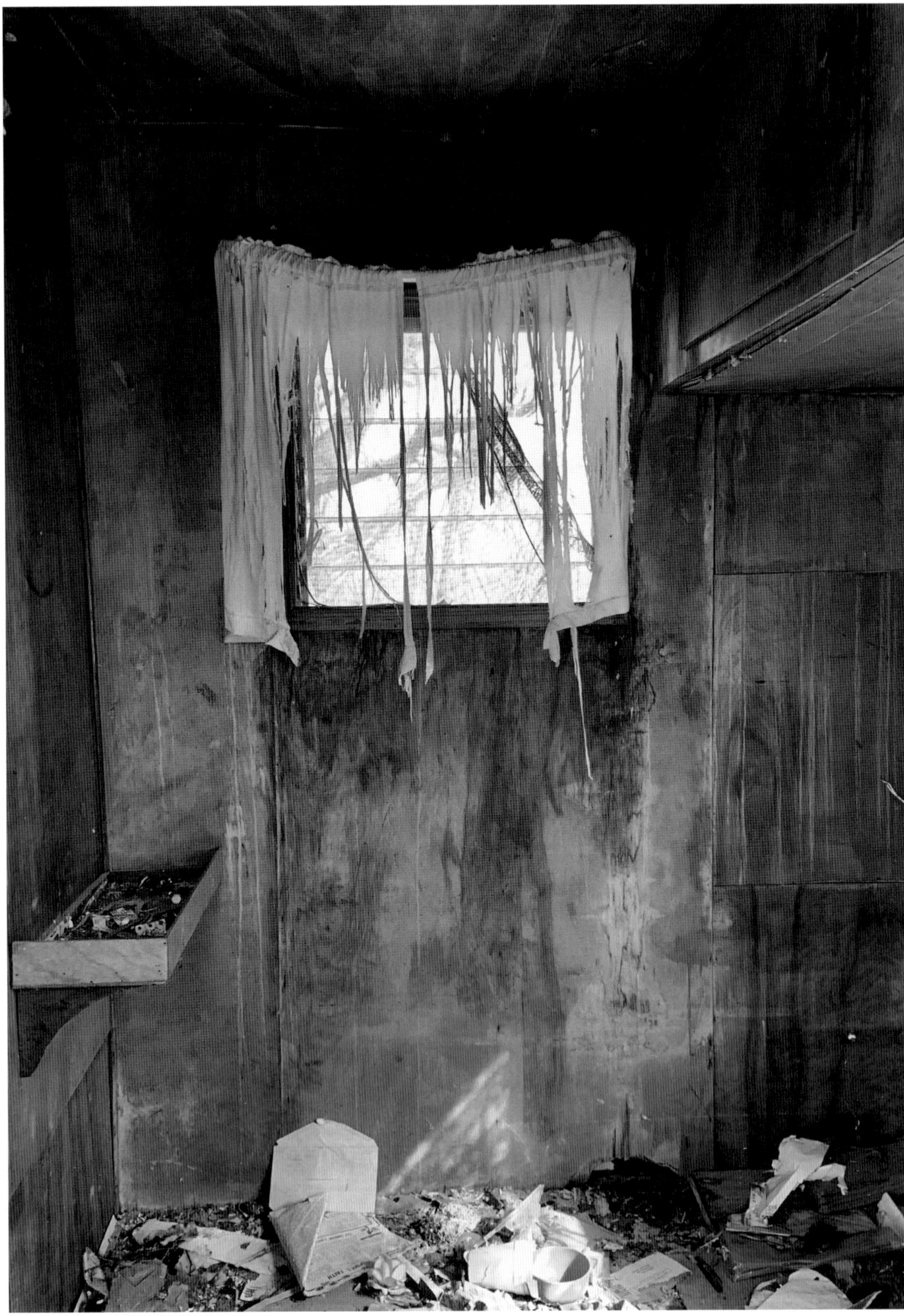

Tattered curtains left blowing in the wind, March 2019.

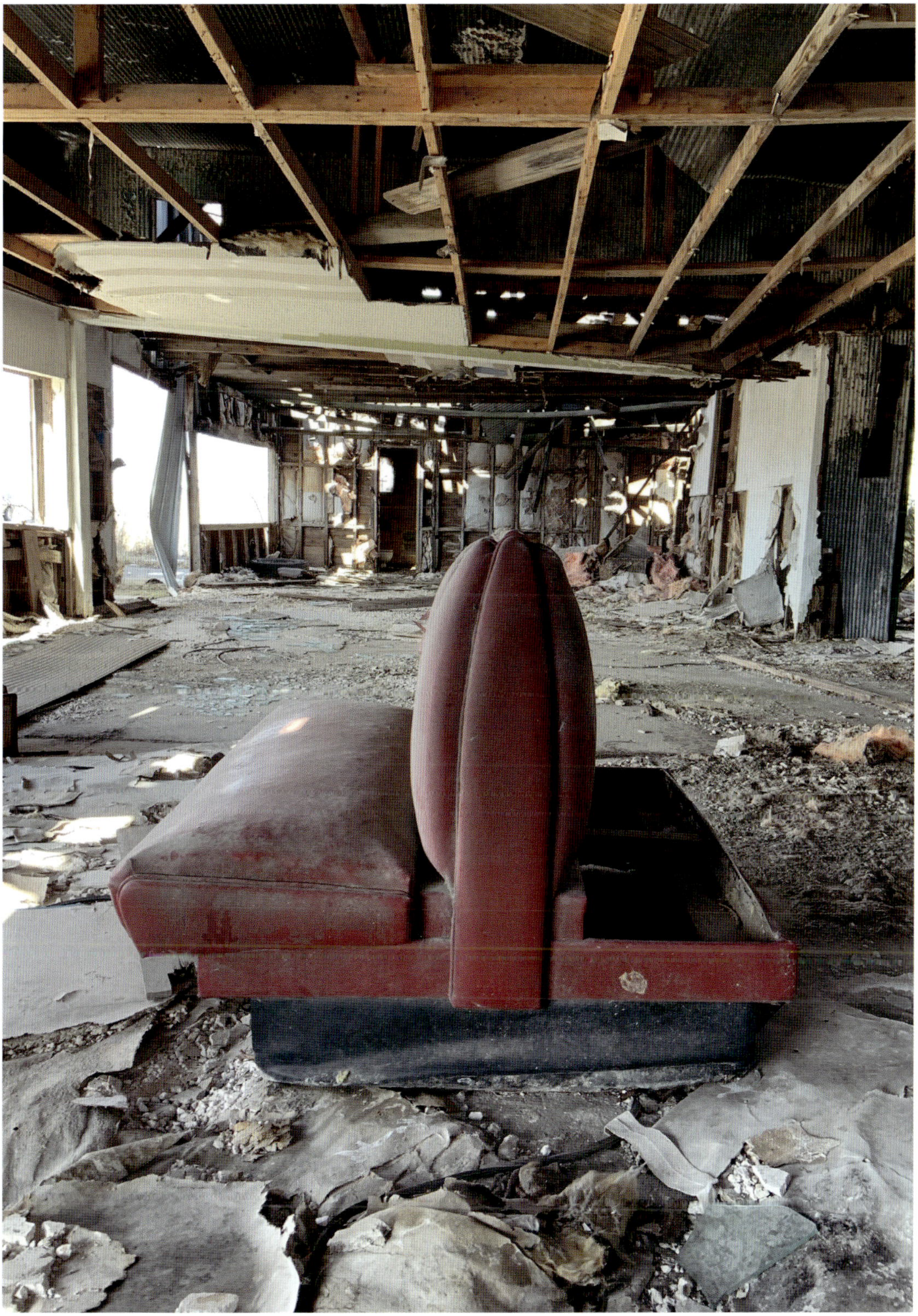

This booth was the only furniture that was left inside the diner, March 2019.

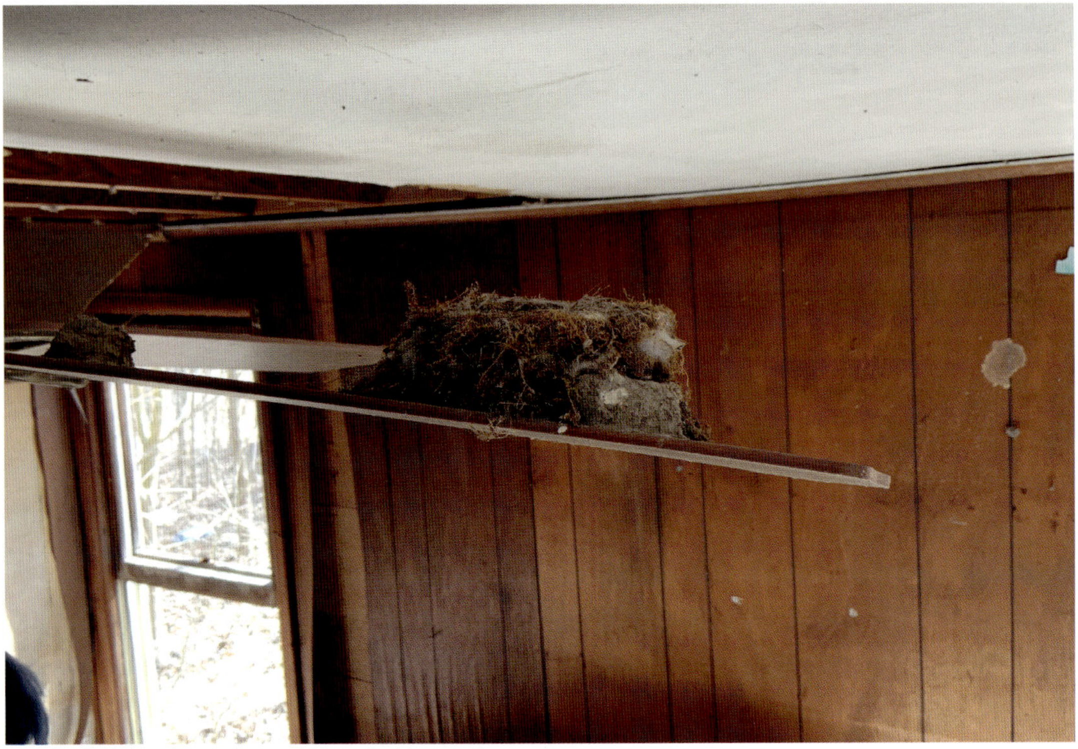

Bird's nest of top of ceiling fan blade in abandoned house, March 2019.

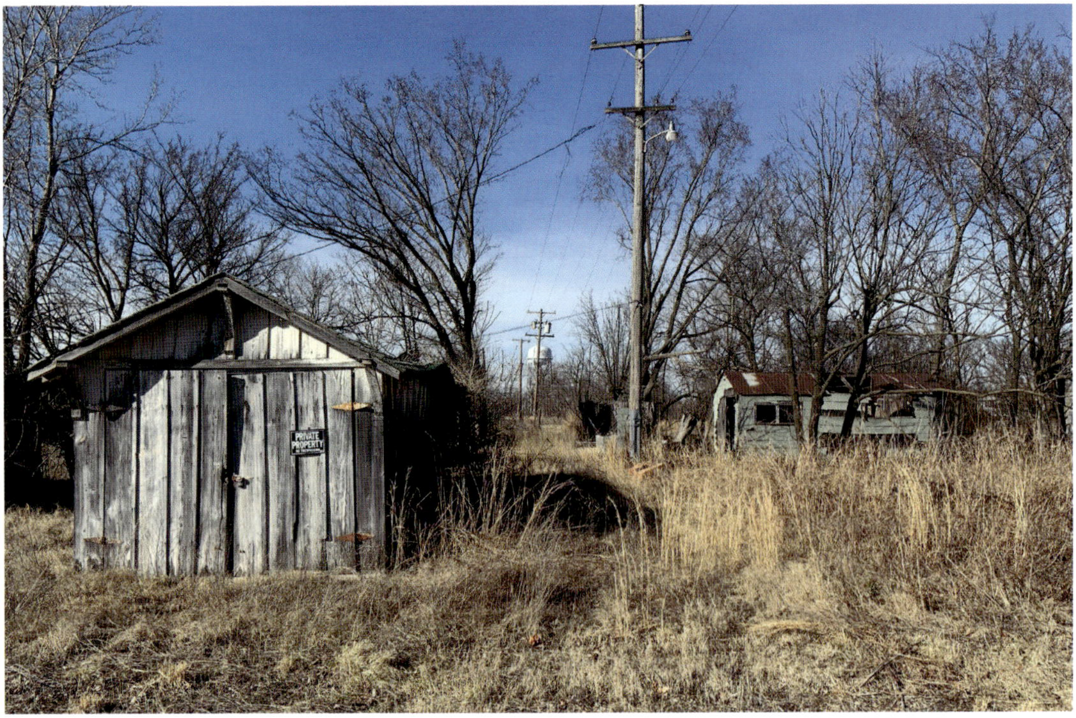

Shed and house behind Claude Best's house, March 2019.

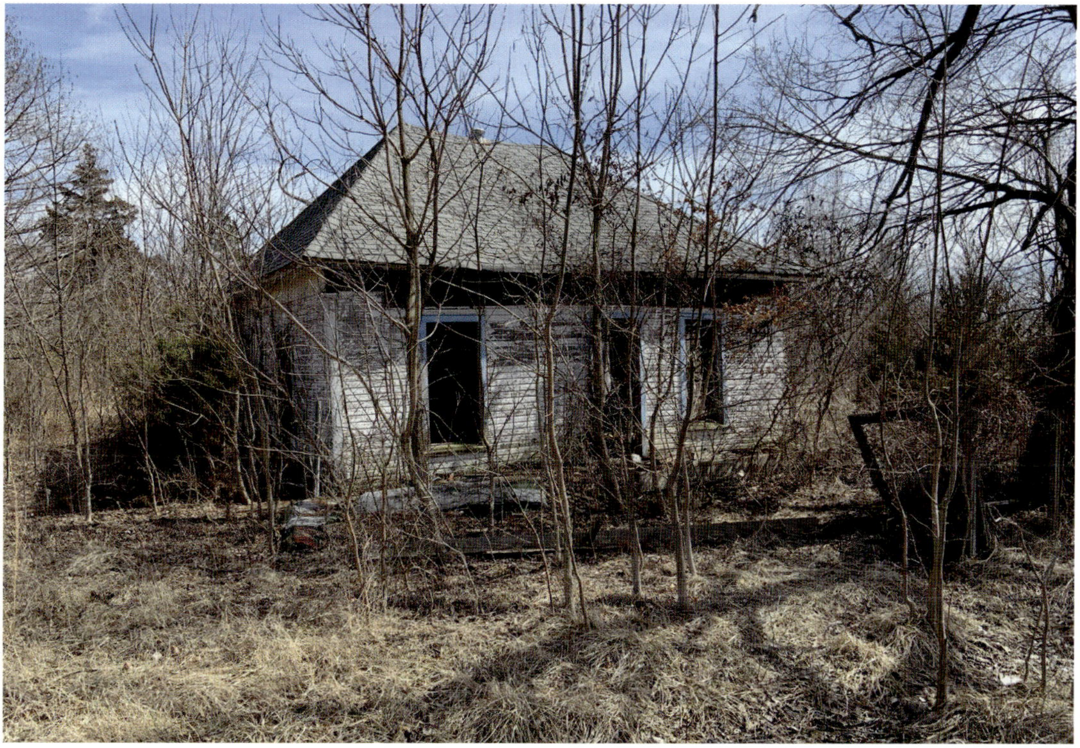

Above: Another house left abandoned, March 2019.

Right: Left side view of the school. One of the many broken windows, probably caused by vandals trying to get into the school, March 2019.

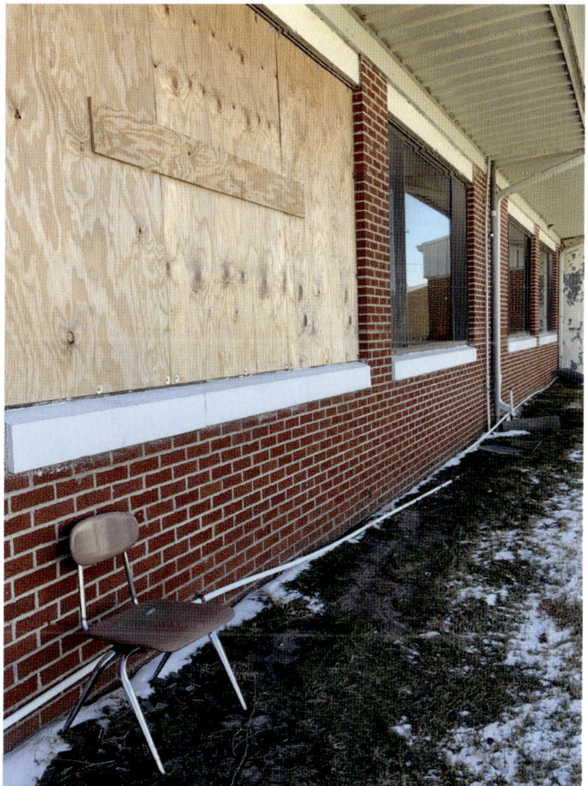

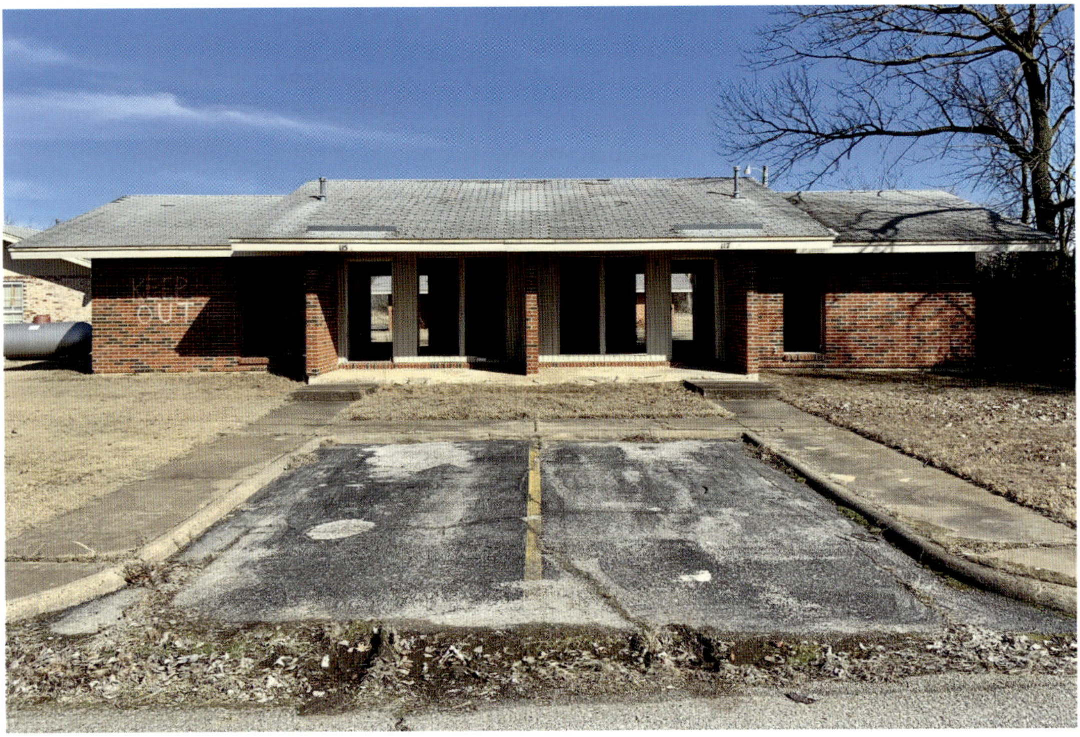

Another building in the complex on Devilliers Circle, March 2019.

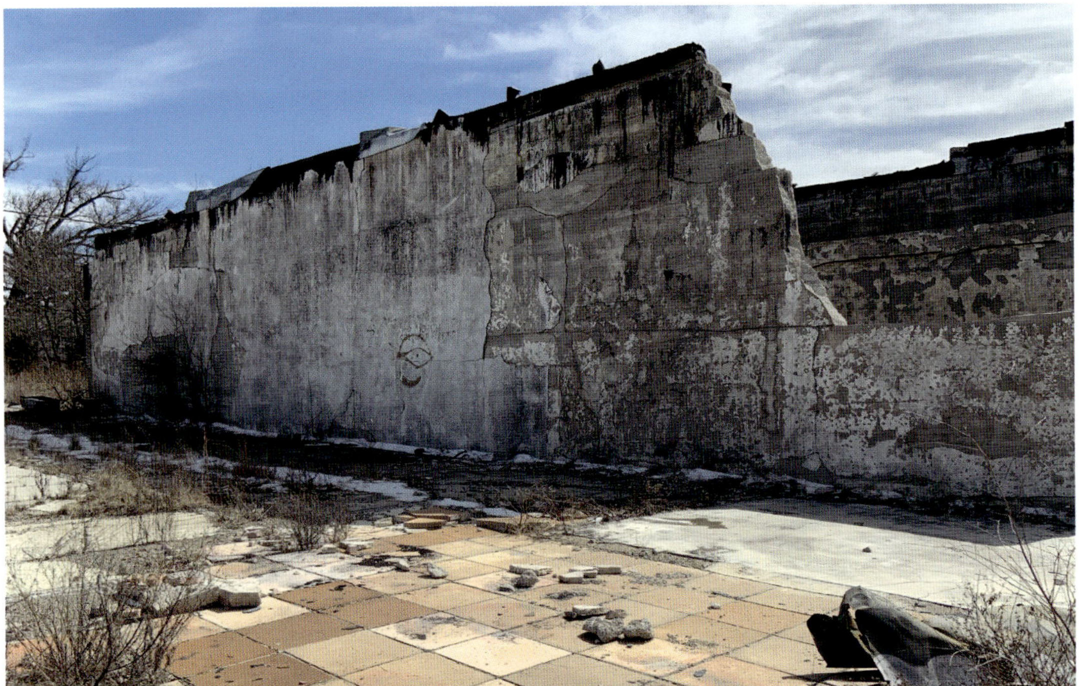

You can still see the tile floor from one of the stores that used to line Connell Avenue, March 2019.

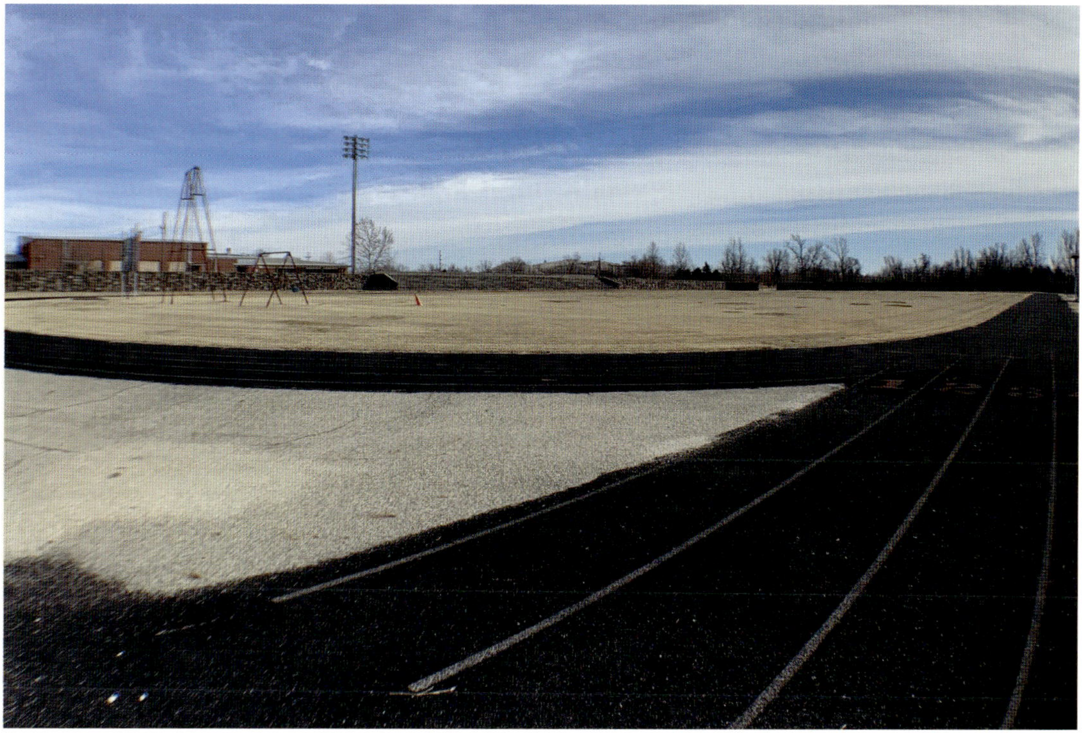

Picher-Cardin's school track. Still in good and maintained condition, March 2019.

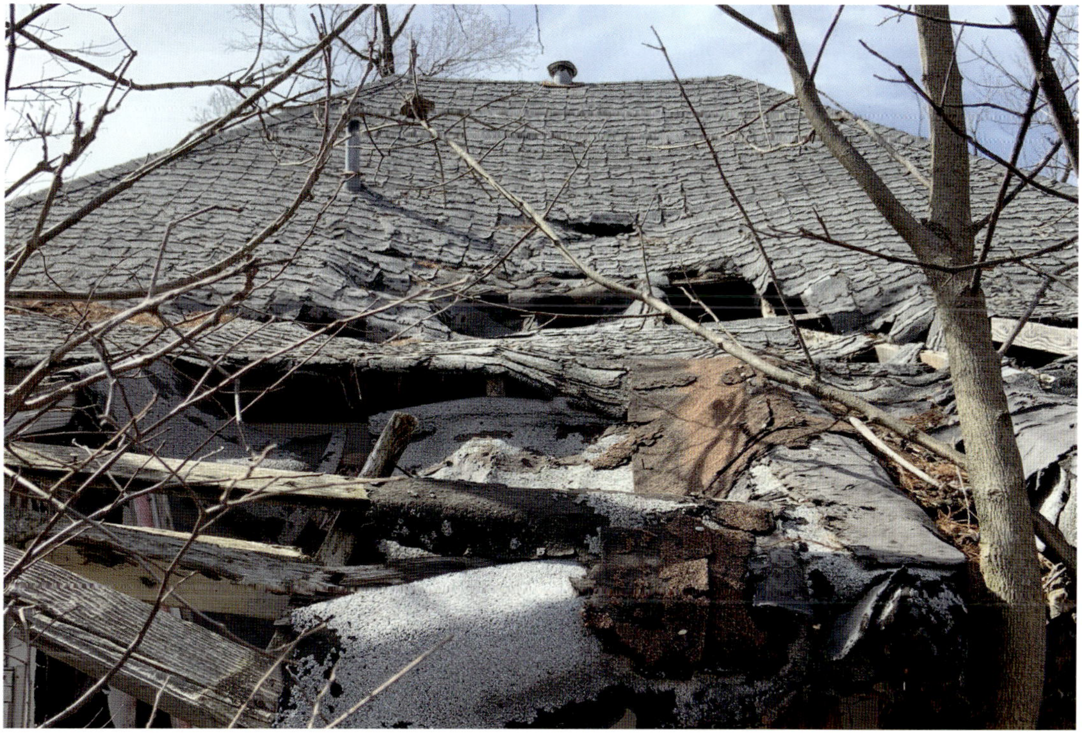

Deteriorating roof on one of the local houses, March 2019.

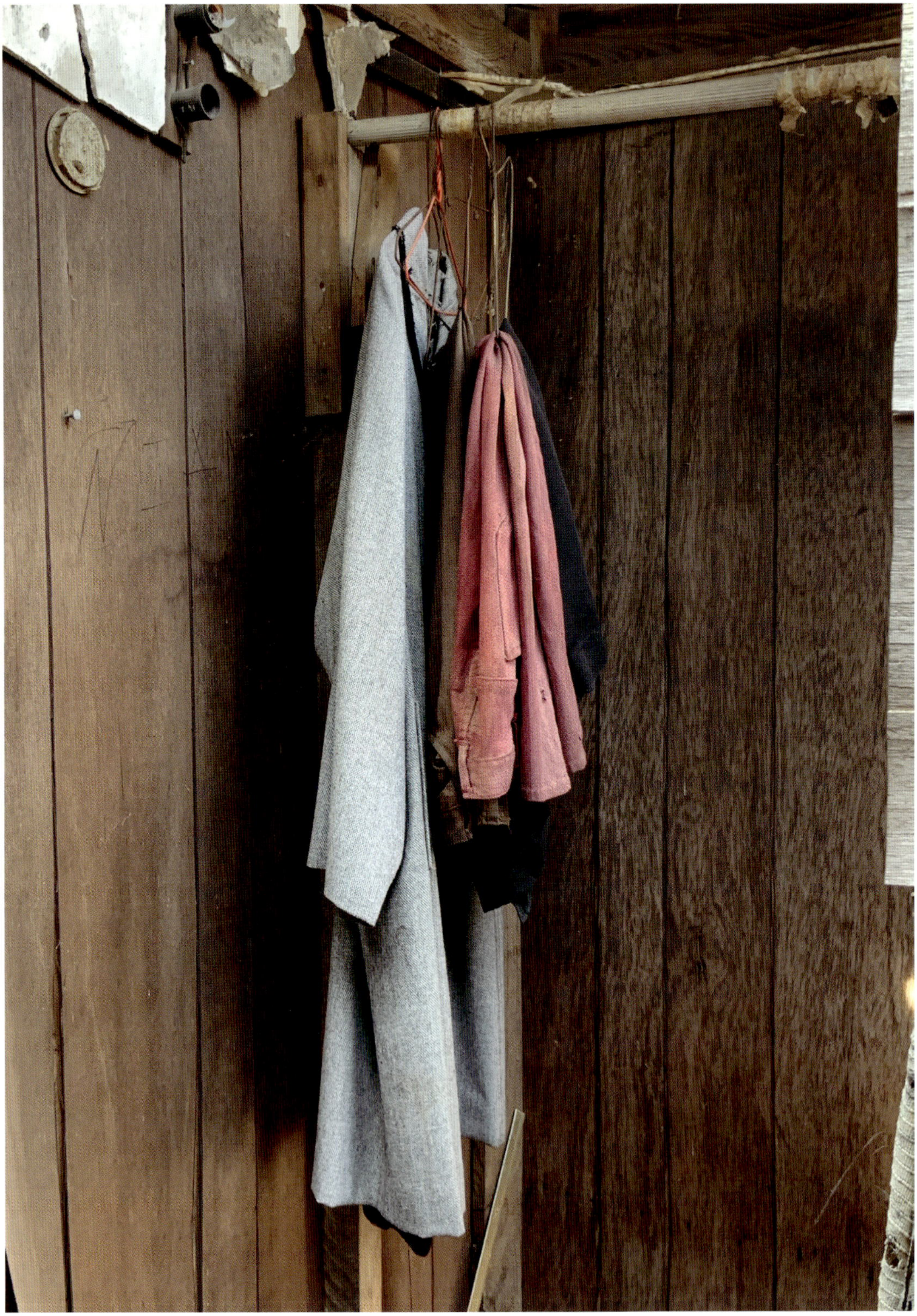

Clothes left hanging in the closet, March 2019.

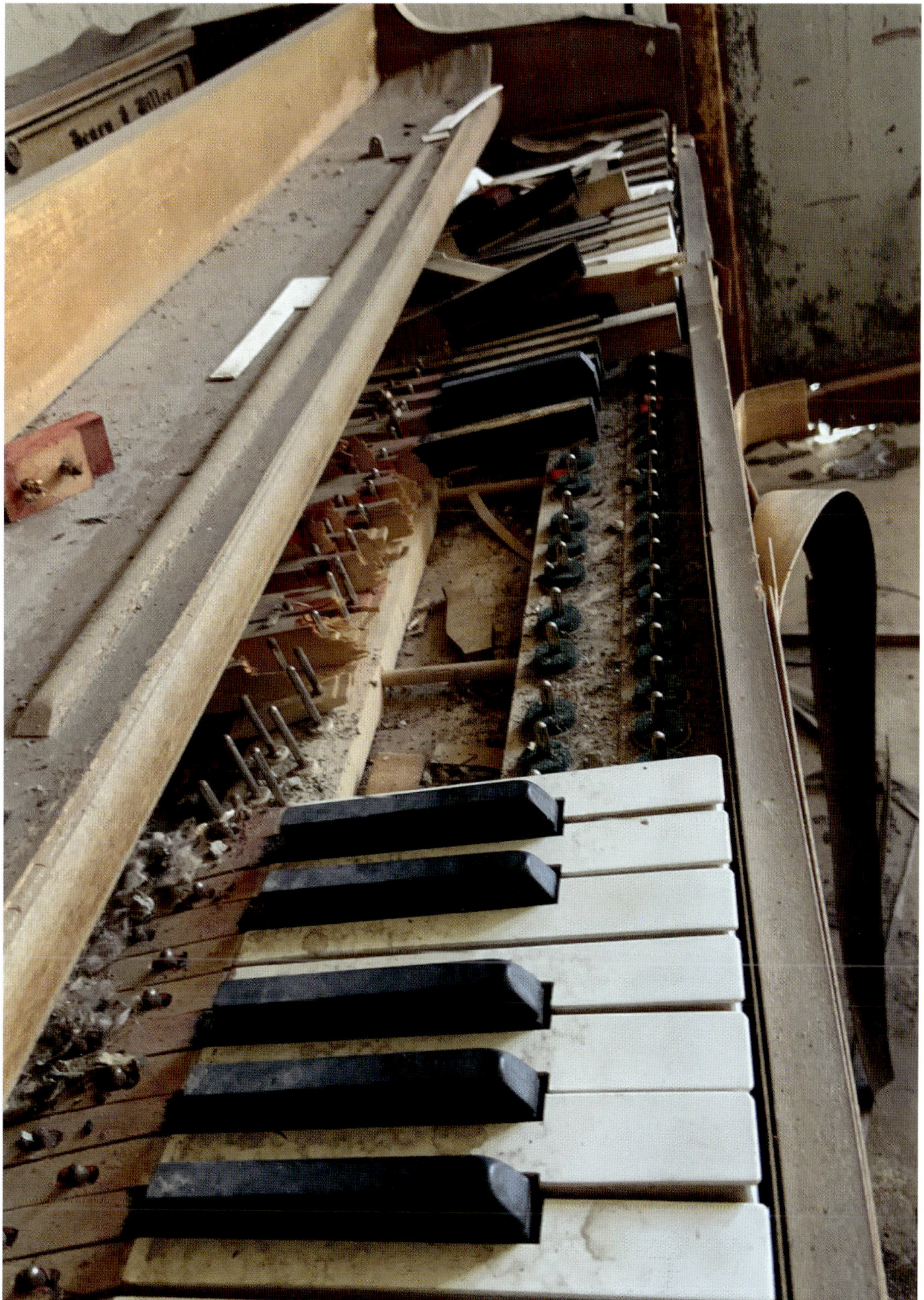

Broken piano found inside Picher Auction house, March 2019.

In late 2010, just over $46 million had already been spent on just relocating the residents, this is not including the last few years of clean up. In 2011, Oklahoma Secretary of the Environment Tyler Powell put the removal of the piles into perspective. He said: "Just removing the chat piles alone could take 30 years if you could move out 100 train car loads each day." Picher's history tells a story that plays out for over a century, and now, if their hypothetical scenario of 100 train cars a day did ever come to fruition, it would still take over another quarter of a century just to remedy the chat piles. Despite this eye-opening perspective, the 2019 EPA Tar Creek Superfund Site strategic plan outlines their progress to date and includes the cleanup plans for the next five years. Part of the completed progress includes 500,000 tons out of chat piles have been sold to "local processors for use." It may not seem like a lot when you look at the grand scheme of things, but every chipping away a mountain into a molehill starts with numerous small efforts. The negative effects proved to have a negative trickle-down effect, but on the other hand, the positive results also prove to have the same trickle-down effect. With nearly 900 acres of land cleared and ready for future use, the reduction of chat, replacing of tainted soil, comes a decrease in the amount of lead effecting the children of the area. Once again, all steps in the right direction. The road back to revitalization will be long and arduous, but despite the uphill battle that has been being fought since 1983, the EPA and, more importantly, the local Quapaw Nation tribe keep foraging ahead to turn back the hands of Picher's damaged time. It is uncertain when the superfund site will have all phases of the cleanup project complete, but with the past and current undertakings combined, it makes completion of each clean up phase, a more attainable goal.

As for the remaining residents, I am guessing that loyalty and solitude are just two of the fingers of the hand that keeps them living there. I can only hope that what is left of the town's buildings do not fall victim to anymore arson or tornados. May the future efforts do what is best for the environment and those who still call Picher their home.

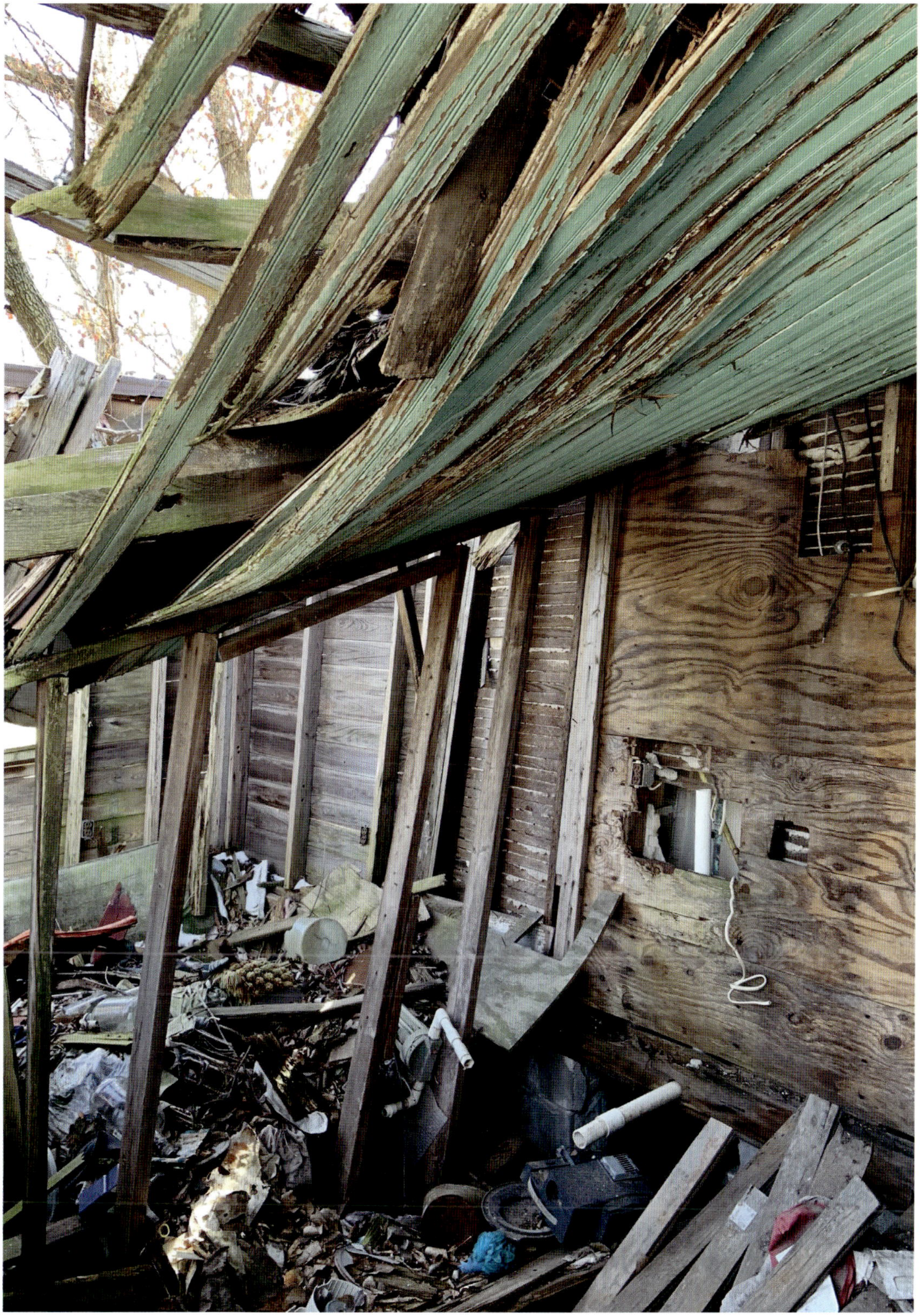

Ceiling collapsing in on back porch area of house, March 2019.

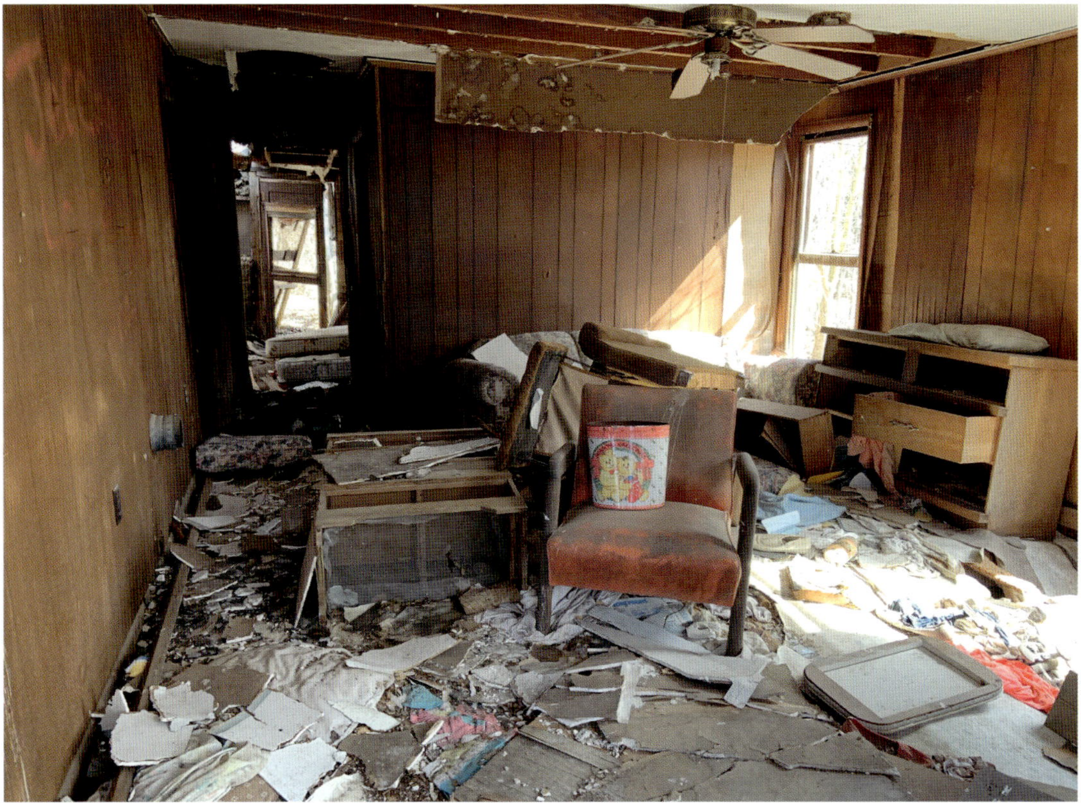

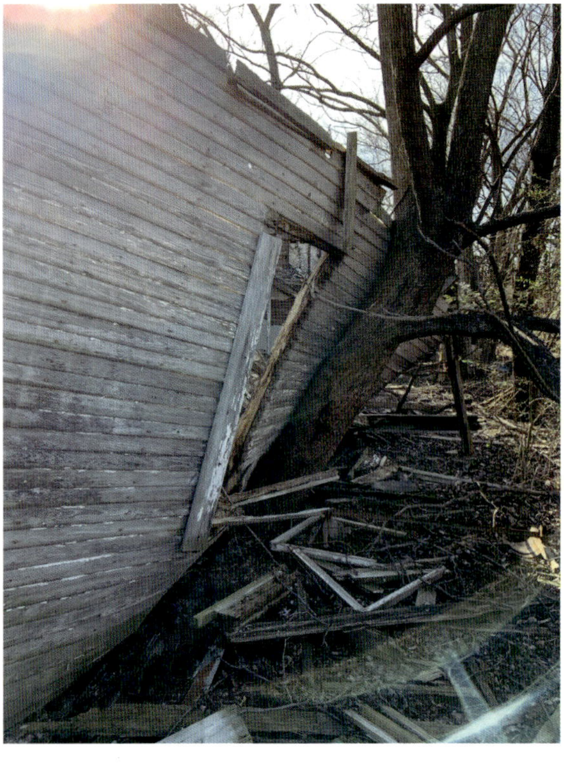

Above: A lot of personal documents and family photos are scattered all over this living room, March 2019.

Left: Side of the house starting to fall over on a tree, March 2019.

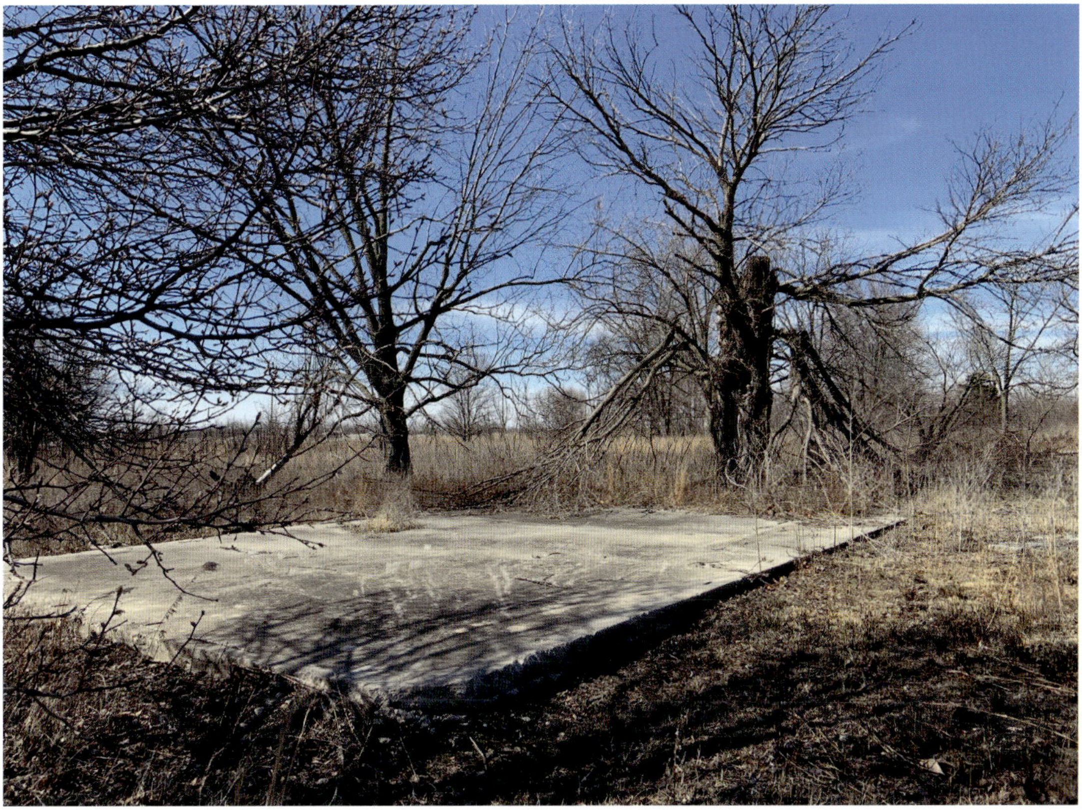

Above: Another foundation slab where a home used to be, March 2019.

Right: Back door of the Full Gospel Revival Church, March 2019.

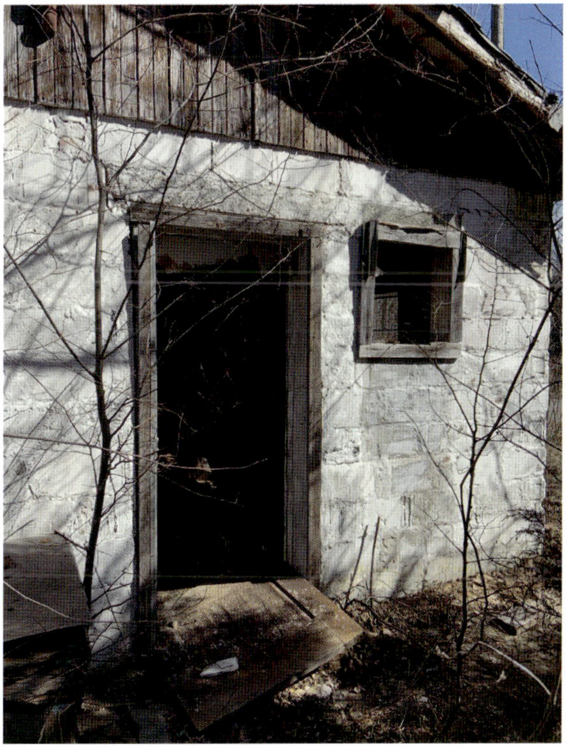

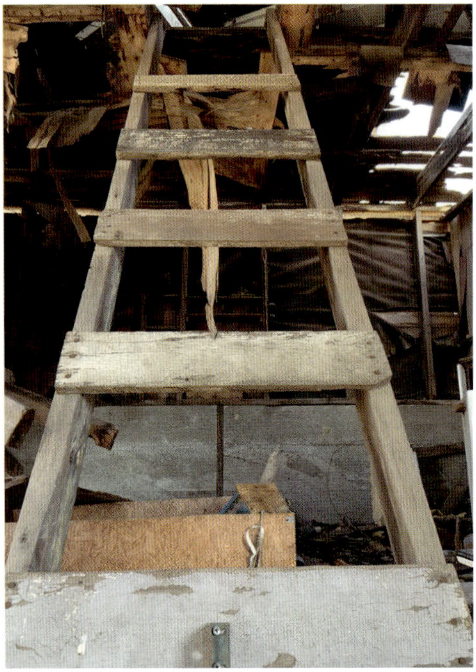

Left: Ladder inside a dilapidated garage, March 2019.

Below: Empty garage left falling apart, March 2019.

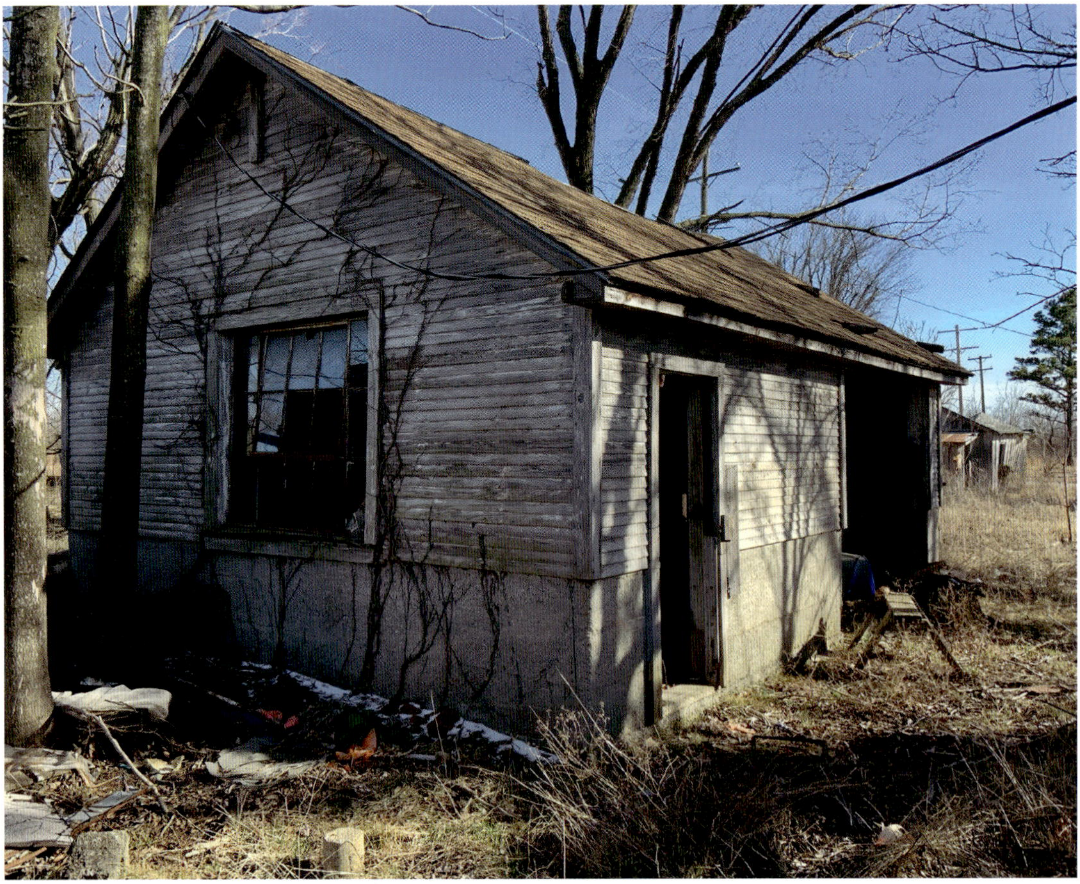

BIBLIOGRAPHY

Center for Disease Control and Prevention, "Lead Poisoning in Children," February 15, 2011.

Environmental Protection Agency, "Tar Creek Ottawa County, OK Cleanup Activities," October 23, 2018.

Environmental Protection Agency, "Tar Creek Superfund Site Strategic Plan: Cleanup Progress & Plans for the Future," 2019.

Estes, A., "Cherokee Nation and Tar Creek," *The Center for Hazardous Substances Research, Kansas State University.*

Everett, D., "Tri-State Lead and Zinc District," *The Encyclopedia of Oklahoma History and Culture. Oklahoma Historical Society.*

Gillham, O. & Stogsdill, S., "Picher School says farewell to last 11," *The Oklahoman*, May 17, 2009.

Gould-Solowat, R. A., "Lead and Pregnancy Know the Risks," *Poison Control*, National Capital Poison Center.

Lewis, G., "Picher, Oklahoma. The biggest environmental disaster you've never heard of," KFSM 5News. November 2, 2015.

Marble, S., "Gary Linderman dies at age 60; 'last man standing' in toxic Oklahoma town," *Los Angeles Times*, June 10, 2015.

Mathews, C. A. & Wood, F., "Picher," *The Encyclopedia of Oklahoma History and Culture.* Oklahoma Historical Society.

Omer, G., "Tar Creek Superfund Site Requires Much More Cleanup, Money," *Tulsa World.* September 27, 2011.

Saulny, S., "Welcome to Our Town. Wish We Weren't Here," *New York Times.* September 13, 2009.

Shepard, D., "Last Residents of Picher, Oklahoma Won't Give Up the Ghost (Town)," *NBC News.* April 26, 2014.

Stogsdill, S., "Fire destroys Picher Mining Field Museum," *Tulsa World.* April 16, 2015

United States Census Bureau, "Picher Oklahoma Demographic Profile Data."

UNKNOWN, "Picher timeline: A history riddled with hardships," *Tulsa World.* January 25, 2011.

ABOUT THE AUTHOR

Regina Daniel received her first camera before the age of ten. From that gift, her passion for photography was born. While on her path of turning that passion into a craft, Regina discovered urban exploration. That discovery would inspire a photo journey to visually immortalize the remnants of what a city leaves behind for bigger and better pursuits.

Regina started and operates Red Vixen's Photography, where she also specializes in architectural and cityscape photography, traveling outside her hometown of Kansas City, Missouri, whenever an abandoned destination calls for it.

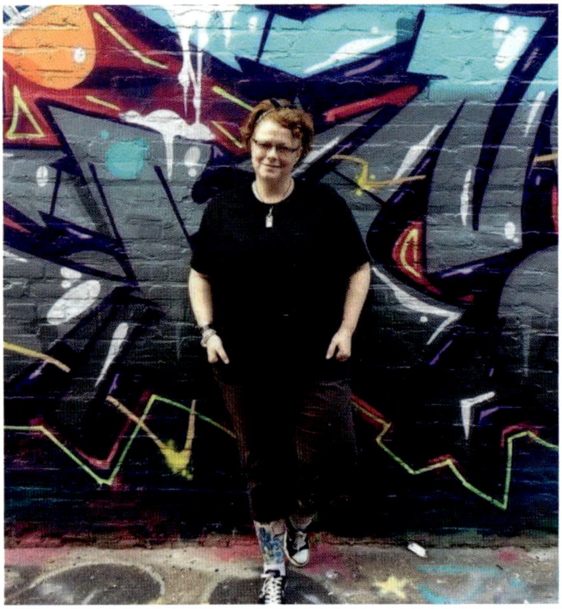